MENTAL ILLNESSES AND TREATMENTS

MENTAL HEALTH OF CHILDREN AND ADULTS IN THE UNITED STATES

SELECT SURVEILLANCE EFFORTS AND DATA

MENTAL ILLNESSES AND TREATMENTS

Additional books in this series can be found on Nova's website under the Series tab.

Additional E-books in this series can be found on Nova's website under the E-book tab.

PUBLIC HEALTH IN THE 21ST CENTURY

Additional books in this series can be found on Nova's website under the Series tab.

Additional E-books in this series can be found on Nova's website under the E-book tab.

MENTAL ILLNESSES AND TREATMENTS

MENTAL HEALTH OF CHILDREN AND ADULTS IN THE UNITED STATES

SELECT SURVEILLANCE EFFORTS AND DATA

GEORGE H. JACKSON
EDITOR

New York

For permission to use material from this book please contact us:
Telephone 631-231-7269; Fax 631-231-8175
Web Site: http://www.novapublishers.com

Library of Congress Cataloging-in-Publication Data

ISBN: 978-1-62808-626-3

Published by Nova Science Publishers, Inc. † New York

CONTENTS

PREFACE

Mental disorders among children are described as "serious deviations from expected cognitive, social, and emotional development". These disorders are an important public health issue in the United States because of their prevalence, early onset, and impact on the child, family, and community, with an estimated total annual cost of $247 billion. A total of 13%–20% of children living in the United States experience a mental disorder in a given year, and surveillance during 1994–2011 has shown the prevalence of these conditions to be increasing. Mental illnesses account for a larger proportion of disability in developed countries than any other group of illnesses, including cancer and heart disease. In 2004, an estimated 25% of adults in the United States reported having a mental illness in the previous year. The economic cost of mental illness in the United States is substantial, approximately $300 billion in 2002. Population surveys and surveys of health-care use measure the occurrence of mental illness, associated risk behaviors (e.g., alcohol and drug abuse) and chronic conditions, and use of mental health–related care and clinical services. This book summarizes data from selected CDC surveillance systems that measure the prevalence and impact of mental illness in the U.S. child and adult populations.

Chapter 1 – Mental disorders among children are described as "serious deviations from expected cognitive, social, and emotional development" (US Department of Health and Human Services Health Resources and Services Administration, Maternal and Child Health Bureau. Mental health: A report of the Surgeon General. Rockville, MD: US Department of Health and Human Services, Substance Abuse and Mental Health Services Administration, Center for Mental Health Services, and National Institutes of Health, National Institute of Mental Health; 1999). These disorders are an important public health issue in the United States because of their prevalence, early onset, and impact on the child, family, and community, with an estimated total annual cost of $247 billion. A total of 13%–20% of children living in the United States experience a mental disorder in a given year, and surveillance during 1994–2011 has shown the prevalence of these conditions to be increasing. Suicide, which can result from the interaction of mental disorders and other factors, was the second leading cause of death among children aged 12–17 years in 2010. Surveillance efforts are critical for documenting the impact of mental disorders and for informing policy, prevention, and resource allocation. This report summarizes information about ongoing federal surveillance systems that can provide estimates of the prevalence of mental disorders and indicators of mental health among children living in the United States, presents estimates of childhood mental disorders and indicators from these systems during 2005–2011, explains limitations, and identifies gaps in information while presenting strategies to bridge those gaps.

Attention-deficit/hyperactivity disorder (6.8%) was the most prevalent parent-reported current diagnosis among children aged 3–17 years, followed by behavioral or conduct problems (3.5%), anxiety (3.0%), depression (2.1%), autism spectrum disorders (1.1%), and Tourette syndrome (0.2% among children aged 6–17 years). An estimated 4.7% of adolescents aged 12–17 years reported an illicit drug use disorder in the past year, 4.2% had an alcohol abuse disorder in the past year, and 2.8% had cigarette dependence in the past month. The overall suicide rate for persons aged 10–19 years was 4.5 suicides per 100,000 persons in 2010. Approximately 8% of adolescents aged 12–17 years reported ≥14 mentally unhealthy days in the past month.

Future surveillance of mental disorders among children should include standard case definitions of mental disorders to ensure comparability and reliability of estimates across surveillance systems, better document the prevalence of mental disorders among preschool-age children, and include additional conditions such as specific anxiety disorders and bipolar disorder. Standard surveillance case definitions are needed to reliably categorize and count mental disorders among surveillance systems, which will provide a more complete picture of the prevalence of mental disorders among children. More comprehensive surveillance is needed to develop a public health approach that will both help prevent mental disorders and promote mental health among children.

Chapter 2 – Mental illnesses account for a larger proportion of disability in developed countries than any other group of illnesses, including cancer and heart disease. In 2004, an estimated 25% of adults in the United States reported having a mental illness in the previous year. The economic cost of mental illness in the United States is substantial, approximately $300 billion in 2002. Population surveys and surveys of health-care use measure the occurrence of mental illness, associated risk behaviors (e.g., alcohol and drug abuse) and chronic conditions, and use of mental health–related care and clinical services. Population-based surveys and surveillance systems provide much of the evidence needed to guide effective mental health promotion, mental illness prevention, and treatment programs.

This report summarizes data from selected CDC surveillance systems that measure the prevalence and impact of mental illness in the U.S. adult population. CDC surveillance systems provide several types of mental health information: estimates of the prevalence of diagnosed mental illness from self-report or recorded diagnosis, estimates of the prevalence of symptoms associated with mental illness, and estimates of the impact of mental illness on health and well-being. Data from the CDC 2005–2008 National Health and Nutrition Examination Survey indicate that 6.8% of adults had moderate to severe depression in the 2 weeks before completing the survey. State-specific data from the CDC 2006 Behavioral Risk Factor Surveillance System (BRFSS), the most recent BRFSS data available, indicate that the prevalence of moderate to severe depression was generally higher in southeastern states compared with other states. Two other CDC surveys on ambulatory care services, the National Ambulatory Medical Care Survey and the National Hospital Ambulatory Medical Care Survey, indicate that during 2007–2008, approximately 5% of ambulatory care visits involved patients with a diagnosis of a mental health disorder, and most of these were classified as depression, psychoses, or anxiety disorders.

Future surveillance should pay particular attention to changes in the prevalence of depression both nationwide and at the state and county levels. In addition, national and state-level mental illness surveillance should measure a wider range of psychiatric conditions and should include anxiety disorders. Many mental illnesses can be managed successfully, and increasing access to and use of mental health treatment services could substantially reduce the associated morbidity.

In: Mental Health of Children and Adults … ISBN: 978-1-62808-626-3
Editor: George H. Jackson

Chapter 1

MENTAL HEALTH SURVEILLANCE AMONG CHILDREN — UNITED STATES, 2005-2011*

Ruth Perou, Rebecca H. Bitsko, Stephen J. Blumberg, Patricia Pastor, Reem M. Ghandour, Joseph C. Gfroerer, Sarra L. Hedden, Alex E. Crosby, Susanna N. Visser, Laura A. Schieve, Sharyn E. Parks, Jeffrey E. Hall, Debra Brody, Catherine M. Simile, William W. Thompson, Jon Baio, Shelli Avenevoli, Michael D. Kogan and Larke N. Huang

SUMMARY

Mental disorders among children are described as "serious deviations from expected cognitive, social, and emotional development" (US Department of Health and Human Services Health Resources and Services Administration, Maternal and Child Health Bureau. Mental health: A report of the Surgeon General. Rockville, MD: US Department of Health and Human Services, Substance Abuse and Mental Health Services Administration, Center for Mental Health Services, and National Institutes of Health, National Institute of Mental Health; 1999). These disorders are an important public health issue in the United States

* This Morbidity and Mortality Weekly Report, Vol. 62, Supplement No. 2, was released by the Centers for Disease Control and Prevention on May 17, 2013.

because of their prevalence, early onset, and impact on the child, family, and community, with an estimated total annual cost of $247 billion. A total of 13%–20% of children living in the United States experience a mental disorder in a given year, and surveillance during 1994–2011 has shown the prevalence of these conditions to be increasing. Suicide, which can result from the interaction of mental disorders and other factors, was the second leading cause of death among children aged 12–17 years in 2010. Surveillance efforts are critical for documenting the impact of mental disorders and for informing policy, prevention, and resource allocation. This report summarizes information about ongoing federal surveillance systems that can provide estimates of the prevalence of mental disorders and indicators of mental health among children living in the United States, presents estimates of childhood mental disorders and indicators from these systems during 2005–2011, explains limitations, and identifies gaps in information while presenting strategies to bridge those gaps.

Attention-deficit/hyperactivity disorder (6.8%) was the most prevalent parent-reported current diagnosis among children aged 3–17 years, followed by behavioral or conduct problems (3.5%), anxiety (3.0%), depression (2.1%), autism spectrum disorders (1.1%), and Tourette syndrome (0.2% among children aged 6–17 years). An estimated 4.7% of adolescents aged 12–17 years reported an illicit drug use disorder in the past year, 4.2% had an alcohol abuse disorder in the past year, and 2.8% had cigarette dependence in the past month. The overall suicide rate for persons aged 10–19 years was 4.5 suicides per 100,000 persons in 2010. Approximately 8% of adolescents aged 12–17 years reported $\geq$14 mentally unhealthy days in the past month.

Future surveillance of mental disorders among children should include standard case definitions of mental disorders to ensure comparability and reliability of estimates across surveillance systems, better document the prevalence of mental disorders among preschool-age children, and include additional conditions such as specific anxiety disorders and bipolar disorder. Standard surveillance case definitions are needed to reliably categorize and count mental disorders among surveillance systems, which will provide a more complete picture of the prevalence of mental disorders among children. More comprehensive surveillance is needed to develop a public health approach that will both help prevent mental disorders and promote mental health among children.

INTRODUCTION

Mental health in childhood is characterized by the achievement of development and emotional milestones, healthy social development, and effective coping skills, such that mentally healthy children have a positive quality of life and can function well at home, in school, and in their communities [1–3]. In this report, children are defined as persons aged <18 years, and adolescents are persons aged 12–17 years. In children, mental disorders are described as “serious deviations from expected cognitive, social, and emotional development” [4] and include conditions meeting criteria described by the Diagnostic and Statistical Manual of Mental Disorders, 4th edition, Text Revision (DSM-IV-TR) [5] or the International Classification of Diseases (ICD) [6,7]. Recently the term mental, emotional, or behavioral disorders has been used to refer to diagnosed mental or substance use disorders [6].

Mental disorders among children are an important public health issue because of their prevalence, early onset, and impact on the child, family, and community. A total of 13%–20% of children living in the United States experience a mental disorder in a given year [6,8–10]. Suicide, which can result from the interaction of mental disorders and other factors, was the second leading cause of death among children aged 12–17 years in 2010 [11]. In the United States, the cost (including health care, use of services such as special education and juvenile justice, and decreased productivity) of mental disorders among persons aged <24 years in the United States was estimated at $247 billion annually [6,12,13]. In 2006, mental disorders were among the most costly conditions to treat in children [14].

Two recent studies have reported substantial increases in use of services for mental disorders among children. One study included insurance claims from approximately 20% of the privately insured U.S. population aged <65 years with private insurance and weighted the data to reflect a national estimate. This study reported a 24% increase in inpatient mental health and substance abuse admissions among children during 2007–2010, as well as increases in use and cost of these services and psychotropic medications for teenagers specifically over the same period [15]. A second nationally representative study, which used data on principal diagnoses for hospital stays in the United States from the Healthcare Cost and Utilization Project, reported that in 2010, mood disorders were among the most common principal diagnoses for all hospital stays among children in the United States, and the rate of hospital stays among children for mood disorders increased 80% during 1997–2010, from 10 to 17 stays per 10,000 population [16].

For some children, mental disorders might result in serious difficulties at home, with peer relationships, and in school [17–19]. These disorders also can be associated with substance use, criminal behavior, and other risk-taking behaviors [20–22]. Persons with mental disorders frequently have more than one type of disorder, with an estimated 40% of children with one mental disorder having at least one other mental disorder [23– 26]. Children with mental disorders also more often have other chronic health conditions (e.g., asthma, diabetes, and epilepsy) than children without mental disorders (6,26–30). Finally, mental disorders in children are associated with an increased risk for mental disorders in adulthood [6], which are associated with decreased productivity, increased substance use and injury, and substantial costs to the individual and society [31,32].

This report, which complements a 2011 report that focused on CDC surveillance of mental illness among adults in the United States [31], describes ongoing independent federal surveillance systems, each addressing different health issues and varying populations, that are used to estimate the prevalence of mental disorders and indicators of mental health among children in the United States and highlights selected national prevalence estimates. Availability of state-based estimates is noted in the surveillance descriptions and tables. Surveillance data from multiple federal agencies, including CDC, the Health Resources and Services Administration (HRSA), and the Substance Abuse and Mental Health Services Administration (SAMHSA), are included. Mental health conditions included in this report include those covered in DSM-IV-TR for which there were recent or ongoing surveillance data collected, including attention-deficit/hyperactivity disorder (ADHD), disruptive behavioral disorders such as oppositional defiant disorder (ODD) and conduct disorder, autism spectrum disorders (ASDs), mood and anxiety disorders including depression, tic disorders, and substance use disorders. Although some consider substance use disorders to be a group of disorders that is distinct from mental disorders, this report refers to substance use disorders as they are referred to in DSM-IV-TR and within the Institute of Medicine (IOM) definition of mental, emotional, and behavioral disorders [5,6]. Selected indicators of mental health, including mentally unhealthy days and suicide, also were assessed.

Surveillance of Mental Disorders Among Children

Public health surveillance involves systematic and ongoing collection ofdata followed by the interpretation and dissemination of the data to encourage public health action [33–35]. Surveillance is critical for policy and program development, documenting the impact of mental disorders among children, tracking changes over time, understanding mental disorders across the lifespan, monitoring health service use and availability [36], increasing prevention and promotion activities, and supporting allocation of funding for services [6,37].

Methods used by different surveillance systems often vary because of the differing priorities of the agencies collecting the data and because of budget constraints. For example, systems vary in terms of 1) what is measured (e.g., diagnostic criteria for a mental disorder, reports of previously diagnosed conditions, reports of mental health symptoms, or other indicators of mental health problems), 2) sample (e.g., age range, oversampling, and geographical coverage), 3) source of the information (e.g., proxy respondent for the child, self-report by the child, or administrative records), 4) the way the data are collected (e.g., in-person interview, telephone interview, self-administered survey, and administrative records), 5) sample size (precision of estimates), and 6) periodicity of data collection (annual or other). Differences in these surveillance modalities and methods might limit comparisons of estimates between different systems [38]. In addition, changes in the characteristics of the same surveillance system over time might limit information about time trends in the prevalence of mental disorders. Information on mental health is collected through independent surveillance systems with varying objectives.

Federal Surveillance Systems, Surveys, and Other Information Systems that Measure Prevalence of Mental Disorders and Indicators of Mental Health Among Children

Childhood mental disorders are not typically the sole focus of federal public health surveillance but are included within systems that address multiple health issues. One exception is the National Comorbidity Survey Replication Adolescent Supplement (NCS-A), a nationally representative population-based prevalence study that was conducted during 2001–2004 and funded by the National Institutes of Mental Health (NIMH) [25,39,40]. Although NCS-A is not an ongoing surveillance system, the survey provided important data on mental disorders among children and was used to calculate national prevalence estimates of several conditions that are not included in current federal surveillance systems. Therefore, survey data from NCS-A, although not current, remain important and relevant and are referenced throughout this report. This report includes descriptions of current, ongoing independent federal surveillance systems that monitor child mental disorders and related mental health indicators (Table 1).

Autism and Developmental Disabilities Monitoring Network

The Autism and Developmental Disabilities Monitoring (ADDM) network is an active surveillance system that has been conducted by CDC since 2000 to estimate the prevalence of ASDs and describe other characteristics among children with ASDs (available at http://www.cdc.gov/ncbddd/autism/addm.html). Fourteen population-based sites in the United States participate in ADDM. The study population in each site includes children aged 8 years during a given surveillance year whose parents or guardians live in the designated geographic region for that site. ADDM focuses on children aged 8 years because a baseline study conducted by CDC demonstrated that the prevalence of autism among children aged 3–10 years is highest in children aged 8 years [41]. A common method is used at each ADDM site. Health and education records are requested from medical providers and public schools that conduct developmental evaluations of children. Specifically, records are requested by sites for children who meet the age and residency eligibility criteria and who have an indication of ASD or another developmental concern based on discharge or other diagnostic codes in health records and special education eligibility codes in education records. The selected records are screened, and those with one or more predefined autism-associated triggers (i.e., behaviors) are fully abstracted. Abstracted information includes basic demographics, verbatim developmental assessment reports, and results of psychometric testing. All abstracted evaluations are reviewed by trained clinicians to determine ASD case status [42]. A child is included as meeting the surveillance case definition for ASD if the child displays behaviors (as described on a comprehensive evaluation completed by a qualified professional) consistent with the DSM-IV-TR diagnostic criteria for autistic disorder, pervasive developmental disorder–not otherwise specified (PDD-NOS, including atypical autism), or Asperger's disorder (5). ADDM has collected data on a biennial cycle since 2000, with period prevalence estimates available for even years during 2000–2008. Prevalence estimates of ASD in this report are from the 2008 surveillance year. The 14 ADDM sites that provided data for the 2008 surveillance year included a total population of

337,093 children aged 8 years, which was 8.4% of the total population of children aged 8 years living in the United States in 2008 [43].

National Health and Nutrition Examination Survey

The National Health and Nutrition Examination Survey (NHANES) is a continuous cross-sectional survey of health and nutritional status conducted by CDC. NHANES uses a multistage probability household sampling design to obtain a nationally representative sample of the civilian noninstitutionalized population living in the United States [44]. Data are collected through personal interviews and dietary intakes, biochemical tests, and physical measurements in a mobile examination center (MEC). The conditions and health indicators studied include cardiovascular disease, diabetes, obesity, environmental exposures, infectious diseases and vaccinations, mental health, oral health, osteoporosis, physical fitness, sexually transmitted diseases, dietary supplements, and prescription medications. Data from NHANES are released in 2-year cycles and are available online (http://www.cdc.gov/ nchs/nhanes. htm); some data are restricted from the public files but are available to researchers through the NCHS Research Data Center (available at http://www.cdc.gov/rdc).

During 1999–2004, NHANES included various modules of the 34 diagnostic assessments from the 12-month Diagnostic Interview Schedule for Children (DISC) (version IV) to measure the prevalence of seven mental disorders during the 12 months before the interview (1999–2004: generalized anxiety disorder and panic disorder; 2000–2004: eating disorder, elimination disorders, major depression/dysthymic disorder, attention-deficit disorder or attention-deficit/hyperactivity disorder [ADD/ADHD], and conduct disorder). DISC, a highly structured diagnostic interview that can be conducted by nonclinicians, was initially developed for epidemiologic studies but also has been used in research studies and clinical settings [45]. Adolescents reported on the generalized anxiety disorder, panic disorder, conduct disorder, depression, and eating disorder modules of DISC during the MEC interview. Parents reported for the adolescents on the conduct disorder, depression, eating disorder, ADHD, and elimination disorder DISC modules during a follow-up phone interview.

NHANES has used the nine-item Patient Health Questionnaire (PHQ-9) since 2005 [46,47] to measure depression during a private interview at the MEC; since 2001, a set of four healthy days measures has been used, including a question on the number of mentally unhealthy days. PHQ-9 is a screening instrument with nine questions about depressive symptoms during the past 2 weeks followed by a single question that assesses associated impairment [46,47]. Among children aged 13–17 years, the PHQ-9 (using a cutoff score of ≥11) has an estimated sensitivity of 89.5% and an estimated specificity of 77.5% for detecting children who meet the DSM-IV criteria for major depression on DISC-IV (46). The mentally unhealthy days question asks: "Now thinking about your mental health, which includes stress, depression, and problems with emotions, for how many days during the past 30 days was your mental health not good?" This question has demonstrated content, construct, and criterion validity in adolescents (48–50). The examination and laboratory data collected allow researchers to examine the relationships between depression and health variables not available on other national surveys. Adolescents aged 12–17 years report for themselves on the PHQ-9 and mentally unhealthy days question.

Approximately 5,000 persons of all ages are examined each year. During 1999–2006, adolescents aged 12–19 years were oversampled, providing larger sample sizes. Adolescents aged 12–17 years are included in this report. During 1999– 2006, the average response rate for adolescents was 87% for the household interview and 85% for the examination. Approximately 78% of adolescents completed the private interview during the MEC examination.

National Health Interview Survey

The National Health Interview Survey (NHIS) has been conducted by CDC since 1957 and is the principal source of information on the health of the civilian noninstitutionalized household population of the United States [51] (available at http://www.cdc.gov/nchs/nhis.htm). NHIS data are collected through in-person household interviews among a nationally representative sample. Households are identified through a multistage probability household sampling design with oversampling of blacks, Hispanics, and Asians for a more precise estimation of health characteristics in these populations.

Selected health and demographic information is collected for all household members, including all of the children in households with children. Then one sample child (if any children aged ≤17 years are present) and one sample adult from each family in NHIS are randomly selected. Additional detailed health-related information, including information on mental health, is collected for the sample child. This information is provided by an adult, usually a parent, who is knowledgeable about the child's health.

The interviewed sample for 2011 consisted of 39,509 households with 26,802 children, from which 12,850 sample child interviews were completed. In 2011, the household response rate was 82%, and the completion rate for the sample child component was 92%, yielding a final response rate of 75% for that component.

Since the redesign of the questionnaire in 1997, autism has been routinely assessed by asking the respondent whether a doctor or health professional has ever told them that the child had any of 10 listed conditions, including autism. The NHIS question changed in 2011 to include autism/ASD. These data are not included in this report because they were undergoing reliability assessments when the data were being prepared for the report. ADHD has also been included since 1997. Respondents for children aged 2–17 years have been asked: "Has a doctor or health professional ever told you that [the child] had... attention-deficit/hyperactivity disorder (ADHD) or attention deficit disorder (ADD)?" Additional questions about a recent diagnosis of depression and about recent anxiety or frequent stress were asked in 2007 and 2012. (The 2012 data were not available at the time the report was prepared and therefore are not included.)

The NHIS questionnaire for children also includes small sets of questions for assessing emotional and behavioral problems in children. For children aged 2–3 years, the items were selected from the Child Behavior Checklist (*52*). For children aged 4–17 years, the items were selected from the Strengths and Difficulties Questionnaire (SDQ) [53,54]. A brief version of the SDQ was developed for use in NHIS and consists of five symptom assessment items and one impairment assessment item. This brief version of the SDQ was included in NHIS in 2002 and 2005–2007 and since 2010. The extended version of the SDQ was included in 2001, 2003, and 2004. NHIS data are available to the public online; restricted data are available to researchers through the NCHS Research Data Center (available at http://www.cdc.gov/rdc).

National Survey of Children's Health

The National Survey of Children's Health (NSCH) is a cross-sectional, random-digit–dial population-based telephone survey that collects information on the physical and emotional health of noninstitutionalized children aged ≤17 years and can be used to produce state and national estimates [55] (available at http://www.cdc.gov/nchs/slaits/nsch.htm). Factors that might relate to children's well-being are emphasized, including medical homes (56), family interactions, parental health, school and after-school experiences, and safety of neighborhoods. The survey is funded by HRSA and conducted by CDC as a module of the State and Local Area Integrated Telephone Survey (SLAITS) mechanism that uses the sampling frame of CDC's National Immunization Survey to identify households with children. One child from each household is randomly selected to be the focus of the interview.

NSCH was administered in 2003, 2007, and 2011–2012. A total of 91,642 child-level interviews were completed for the 2007 NSCH; the household screening response rate was 71%, the interview completion rate was 66%, and the overall response rate was 47%. Data were collected from a parent or guardian in the household who was knowledgeable about the health and health care of the randomly selected child. The respondent was the mother (biological, stepmother, foster mother, or adoptive mother) for 73.5% of the children.

The 2007 NSCH assessed the presence of mental health problems or conditions in children aged 2–17 years. Parents or guardians were asked about 1) depression; 2) anxiety problems; 3) behavioral or conduct problems, such as ODD or conduct disorder; 4) autism, Asperger's disorder, pervasive developmental disorder, or other ASDs; 5) developmental delay; 6) Tourette syndrome; and 7) ADD/ADHD. For each condition, parents were asked whether they had ever been told by a doctor or other health-care provider that their child had the condition and whether the child still had the condition. For children with current problems or conditions, parents were asked to rate the severity of their child's condition as mild, moderate, or severe. Parents were also asked whether their children received mental health treatment or counseling or took medications because of a problem with emotions, concentration, or behavior. NSCH data are available to the public online; data from the latest survey (2011–2012) became available in 2013 but were not available for inclusion in this report.

National Survey on Drug Use and Health

The National Survey on Drug Use and Health (NSDUH) is the primary source of statistical information on the use of alcohol, tobacco, illicit drugs, and nonmedical use of prescription drugs in the United States [57] (available at http://www.samhsa.gov/data/NSDUH.aspx). The survey includes several modules of questions that focus on mental health issues.

Conducted by the federal government since 1971 (annually since 1990), NSDUH is sponsored by SAMHSA. NSDUH collects data through in-person household interviews with a representative sample of the noninstitutionalized population. Thus, NSDUH excludes homeless persons who are not in shelters, military personnel on active duty, and residents of institutional group quarters such as prisons and long-term hospitals.

NSDUH is a state and nationally representative survey with approximately 150,000 addresses screened and approximately 70,000 respondents interviewed each year. Adolescents and young adults are oversampled, and each state's sample is approximately equally distributed among three age groups: 12–17 years, 18–25 years, and ≥26 years. In 2011, the weighted response rates were 87% for household screening, 74% for interviewing, and 65% overall.

Data on substance use collected by NSDUH among adolescents aged 12–17 years include information on the recency and frequency of use of tobacco products, alcohol, marijuana, cocaine, heroin, inhalants, and hallucinogens and nonmedical use of prescription drugs. NSDUH collects information on symptoms of substance use disorders in the past year, major depressive episodes (MDEs) during the lifetime and in the past year, and MDEs accompanied by impairment in one or more role domains. The case definitions for substance use disorders and MDEs are based on DSM-IV criteria. Additional information collected for adolescents includes mental health service use, substance use treatment, treatment for depression, risk and protective factors, parental mental illness, and parental substance use. NSDUH also collects respondent reports of anxiety and depression during the lifetime and in the past year as diagnosed by a doctor or medical professional. However, estimates based on these items are not provided in this report, pending the completion of quality assessments. NSDUH data are publicly available (http://www.samhsa.gov/data/NSDUH.aspx).

National Violent Death Reporting System

The National Violent Death Reporting System (NVDRS) is a population-based active surveillance system conducted by CDC that provides a census of violent deaths that occur within participating states (available at http://www.cdc.gov/ncipc/wisqars/NVDRS/About-NVDRS.htm#disclaimer). For the purposes of NVDRS, violence is defined as "the intentional use of physical force or power (threatened or actual) against a person, or against a group or community that either results in, or has a high likelihood of resulting in injury, death, psychological harm, maldevelopment (e.g. arrested physical, mental, intellectual, emotional, or social development) or deprivation" [58]. Violent deaths include child maltreatment deaths, intimate partner homicides and other homicides, suicides, and legal intervention deaths (i.e., when a decedent is killed by a police officer or other person with specified legal authority to use deadly force). Unintentional firearm injury deaths and deaths of undetermined intent also are included in the system.

NVDRS began collecting data in 2003 with seven states participating (Alaska, Maryland, Massachusetts, New Jersey, Oregon, South Carolina, and Virginia); six states joined in 2004 (Colorado, Georgia, North Carolina, Oklahoma, Rhode Island, and Wisconsin), four more joined in 2005 (California, Kentucky, New Mexico, and Utah), and two joined in 2010 (Michigan and Ohio), for a total of 19 states. CDC provides funding for state participation and anticipates that NVDRS will eventually expand to include all 50 states, the District of Columbia (DC), and U.S. territories [59].

NVDRS obtains data from multiple complementary data sources, including death certificates, medical examiner and coroner records, and law enforcement reports. Secondary sources used by some participating states include child fatality review team data, supplementary homicide reports, hospital data, and crime laboratory data. Because NVDRS is an incident-based system, violent incidents can include more than one person and more than one weapon. Individual-level data include manner of death; injury mechanism; whether each individual involved in an incident is a victim, suspect, or both; and circumstances surrounding injury. The circumstance data for homicide, suicide, and undetermined deaths include such factors as mental health history and status (e.g., current depressed mood, current mental health problems, current treatment for mental health problems, whether treatment has ever been received for mental health problems, and history of suicide attempts), whether a victim disclosed the intent to die by suicide, interpersonal conflicts, alcohol or other substance use, and criminal acts. Because no sampling is involved, all identified violent deaths in participating states are included. Data from 2005–2009 are included in this report.

NVDRS data are publicly accessible through CDC's Web-based Injury Statistics Query and Reporting System (WISQARS) [11]. Potentially identifiable NVDRS microdata are also available via a formal request to CDC.

National Vital Statistics System

Mortality statistics from the National Vital Statistics System (NVSS) are based on information from death certificates filed in the 50 states and DC and processed by CDC [60] (available at http://www.cdc.gov/nchs/deaths.htm). Vital statistics mortality data are a fundamental source of demographic, geographic, and cause-of-death information for the United States.

The mortality file includes medical information on cause of death (including suicide) and demographic information on age, sex, race, Hispanic origin, state of residence, and educational attainment. The death registration area for all states and DC has been in existence since 1932. CDC obtains information on deaths from the registration offices of each of the 50 states, New York City, DC, Puerto Rico, the U.S. Virgin Islands, Guam, American Samoa, and the Northern Mariana Islands. Data are sent to CDC through the Vital Statistics Cooperative Program.

The completion and filing of the death certificate with the state vital registrar is the responsibility of the funeral director. The funeral director obtains demographic data for the death certificate from an informant. The physician in attendance at the death is required to certify the cause of death. For suicides and other unnatural causes of death, a coroner or medical examiner typically is required to investigate and certify the cause of death.

All NVSS mortality files have an underlying cause of death for each record. The underlying cause of death is defined as 1) the disease or injury that initiated the train of morbid events leading directly to death or 2) the circumstances of the accident or violence that produced the fatal injury. Beginning with data year 1999, underlying causes of death coded as any of the ICD–10 codes *U03, X60–X84, or Y87.0 result in the death being categorized as a suicide. Data from 2010 are included in this report.

NVSS data are publicly accessible through CDC WONDER [61] and CDC WISQARS [11] (available at http://www.cdc. gov/nchs/deaths.htm). Restricted access to NVSS records for individual cases also are available via a formal request to CDC.

School-Associated Violent Death Surveillance Study

The School-Associated Violent Death Surveillance Study (SAVD), conducted by CDC in collaboration with the U.S. Department of Education and the U.S. Department of Justice, describes the epidemiology of school-associated violent deaths, identifies common features of these deaths, estimates the rate of school-associated violent death in the United States, and identifies potential risk factors for these deaths [62] (available at http://www.cdc.gov/violenceprevention/youthviolence/ schoolviolence/SAVD.html). SAVD includes descriptive data on all identified school-associated violent deaths in the United States, including all homicides, suicides, or legal intervention incidents in which the fatal injury occurred on the campus of a functioning elementary or secondary school, while the victim was on the way to or from regular sessions at such a school, or while the victim was attending or on the way to or from an official school-sponsored event. Victims of such incidents include nonstudents, students, and staff members. Data reported here are restricted to those pertaining to children aged 5–18 years. SAVD includes descriptive information about the school, event, victims, and offenders. Although SAVD attempts to include all school-associated violent deaths, deaths that did not appear in media databases during the case-identification period for specific years and were not identified by supplemental case finding efforts might be missed. In addition, cases that are never reported by the media might be overlooked altogether because case-finding strategies rely heavily on news reports. However, because most of the recognized cases receive extensive, often nationwide, coverage, it is unlikely that many cases of school-associated homicide or suicide went entirely unreported. If any such cases did occur, they might differ from the cases that were deemed more newsworthy and are characterized in this report. SAVD has collected data from July 1, 1992, through the present.

SAVD uses an ongoing four-step process to identify and collect data on school-associated violent deaths: 1) identification through a media search; 2) confirmation with law enforcement officials to determine whether the event meets the case definition; 3) interviews with law enforcement and school officials regarding details about the school, event, victims, and offenders; and 4) request for a copy of the full law enforcement report for each case. Detailed event information is collected for each case including the geographic location of injury, the context of injury (while classes were being held, during break, etc.), motive for injury, method of injury, and school and community events happening around the time period. Information obtained on victims and offenders includes demographics, circumstances of the event (date and time, alcohol or drug use, and number of persons involved), types and origins of weapons, criminal history, psychological risk factors, school-related problems, extracurricular activities, and family history, including structure and stressors.

SAVD currently collects mental health-related information (for victims and offenders) at the time of the event and in the year before the event. At the time of the event, information collected includes demonstration of symptoms consistent with an attention deficit or a hyperactivity disorder (e.g., impulsivity, short attention span, distractibility), whether the victim or offender has a diagnosis of ADHD or another hyperactivity disorder, treatment for ADHD or another hyperactivity disorder, and presence of a diagnosed learning disability. Information assessed for the year before the event includes receipt of school-sponsored psychological counseling services, treatment for depression, presence of thoughts of suicide or threats of suicide, presence of plans for suicide, and previous suicide attempts. Data from July 1, 2005–June 30, 2011, are included in this report.

National Youth Risk Behavior Survey

The national Youth Risk Behavior Survey (YRBS) [63] was developed in the late 1980s to monitor health-risk behaviors that contribute substantially to the leading causes of death, disability, and social problems among children and young adults in the United States (available at http://www.cdc.gov/ yrbs). CDC conducts the national YRBS to monitor priority health-risk behaviors, obesity, and asthma among high school students in the United States.

The national YRBS uses a three-stage cluster sample design to produce a representative sample of public and private high school students in grades 9–12 in the 50 states and DC. The national YRBS has been conducted biennially since 1991. In 2011, a total of 15,425 questionnaires were completed in 158 schools. YRBS questionnaires are self-administered; students record their responses on a computer-scannable booklet or answer sheet. In 2011, the student response rate was 87%, the school response rate was 81%, and the overall response rate was 71%.

The national YRBS assesses several categories of behaviors that are associated with children's mental health, including behaviors that contribute to unintentional injuries and violence, bullying, sexual behavior, body weight, nutrition, and physical activity. Indicators of mental health covered by YRBS include feeling sad or hopeless; tobacco, alcohol, and other drug use; and suicide-related behaviors. One symptom of depression, feeling sad or hopeless, is assessed by the question: "During the past 12 months, did you ever feel so sad or hopeless almost every day for 2 weeks or more in a row that you stopped doing some usual activities?" To assess suicidal ideation and attempts during the past 12 months, adolescents are asked: "Did you ever seriously consider attempting suicide? Did you make a plan about how you would attempt suicide? How many times did you actually attempt suicide? Did any suicide attempt result in an injury, poisoning, or overdose that had to be treated by a doctor or nurse?"

The national YRBS is part of a large surveillance system, the Youth Risk Behavior Surveillance System (YRBSS), which also includes state and local school-based surveys [64]. Data for the national YRBS and the YRBSS are publicly available.

Findings from Surveillance Systems and Surveys and Descriptions of Mental Disorders and Mental Health Indicators

This section presents findings from recent independent federal surveillance systems and surveys that collect data on mental disorders and mental health indicators among children in the United States. A summary of prevalence estimates of childhood mental disorders for which data are not routinely collected (and that are not included in this report) is provided (Table 2). Also provided is a summary of prevalence estimates for which data are routinely collected and that are included in this report (Table 3). Although children are defined as persons aged <18 years, estimates are generally restricted to children aged ≥3 years and <18 years.

Mental Disorders

ADHD, ODD, and Conduct Disorder ADHD

ADHD, ODD, and conduct disorder are a set of behavioral disorders that frequently occur together [65]. ADHD is characterized by developmentally inappropriate levels of inattention, hyperactivity, impulsivity, or a combination of these, which impair functioning in multiple settings [5]. DSM-IV-TR classifies children with ADHD into one of three subtypes corresponding to their symptom profile: predominantly inattentive, predominantly hyperactive and impulsive, or combined. The functional limitations related to ADHD symptoms commonly result in academic, peer, and family problems [5,66,67]. In addition, children with ADHD are more likely to have higher rates of unintentional injuries, emergency department visits, smoking, alcohol use, and illicit substance use [68–75].

Household adults who have knowledge of the child's health status (usually parents) who participated in NHIS were asked whether a doctor or other health-care provider ever told them that the sampled child has ADD or ADHD. The 2003 and 2007 NSCH included the same question. NSCH also included questions about current ADHD and level of severity among children with an ADHD diagnosis. NHANES (2000–2004) assessed ADHD among children aged 8–15 years using parents as respondents to the DISC-IV diagnostic interview.

The prevalence of parents reporting that their child had ever received an ADHD diagnosis among children aged 3–17 years in 2007 was lower on the NHIS (7.6%) than NSCH (8.9%) (Table 3 and Table 4). Differences in the method of data collection (i.e., in-person versus telephone interview), question placement, context, and other survey methods might have affected the estimates. Demographic patterns from the two surveys are consistent, with estimates higher among boys, older children, non-Hispanic children, children living in families in which the most highly educated adult was a high school graduate, children in families with insurance, children in the Midwest and South, and children living in households with incomes ≤100% of the federal poverty level.

Based on DISC-IV (NHANES) data, the estimated prevalence of ADHD in the past 12 months was 8.6% among children aged 8–15 years during 2001–2004 [9], which is very similar to the estimate from NHIS, based on parent report, for children aged 8–15 years during 2001–2004 (8.9%, 95% confidence interval: 8.4–9.3). However, children who meet DISC criteria for ADHD are not necessarily the same population of children who have a parent-reported diagnosis of ADHD [76].

Parents who participated in the 2007 NSCH and reported that their child had ever received a diagnosis of ADHD also were asked whether the child had a current diagnosis of the condition. Based on parent report, the estimated national prevalence of current ADHD among children aged 3–17 years was 6.8% in 2007. Although estimates of parent-reported current ADHD are lower than estimates of ever-diagnosed ADHD, they have a similar demographic pattern (Tables 3 and 4).

Most recently, NHIS data indicate that parents of 8.5% of children aged 3–17 years in 2009–2010 and 8.4% in 2011 had ever been told their child had ADHD. Demographic patterns were similar to those reported above. Based on parent-reported data in 2011, ever having ADHD was more common among boys than girls, increased with age, was higher among those with health insurance than without health insurance and was highest among those with the lowest poverty-income ratio. Prevalence was highest among white non-Hispanic children and black non-Hispanic children and lower among Hispanic children, non-Hispanic "other" children, and non-Hispanic children of multiple races. Prevalence was higher in the South than the West or Northeast and lower in the West than the Midwest. Prevalence did not differ by the highest level of education in the household.

ODD and Conduct Disorder

ODD is characterized by a pattern of developmentally inappropriate, negative, aggressive, and defiant behavior that occurs for ≥6 months [5]. Children with ODD frequently lose their temper, argue with adults, defy or refuse to comply with rules and requests, deliberately annoy others, blame their behavior on others, are easily annoyed, and are spiteful or vindictive. Children with conduct disorder consistently ignore the basic rights of others and violate social norms and rules [5]. To meet DSM-IV criteria for conduct disorder, three or more behaviors (e.g., aggression to persons and animals, destruction of property, deceitfulness or theft, and serious violations of rules) must have been present in the past 12 months, with at least one exhibited in the past 6 months. When occurring with ADHD, ODD and conduct disorder often predict later antisocial personality disorder, psychoactive substance use disorders, smoking, and bipolar disorder [77].

Only NSCH has asked parents to report about these other disruptive behavioral disorders. A question included in the 2007 NSCH asked the parent whether a doctor or other healthcare provider ever told them that the child had behavioral or conduct problems, such as ODD or conduct disorder. Conduct disorder also was previously assessed using parent report of symptoms on DISC-IV in NHANES from 2000–2004.

Parent-reported data from NSCH indicated that 4.6% of children aged 3–17 years had a history of a behavioral or conduct problem such as ODD or conduct disorder. In addition, an estimated 3.5% of children had a current behavioral or conduct problem (Table 3 and Table 5). Prevalence of these disorders was twice as high among boys as among girls (ever had the diagnosis: 6.2% versus 3.0%; current diagnosis: 4.6% versus 2.2%). Reported prevalence increased with age, from a low of 1.3% among children aged 3–5 years age to a high of 4.2% among children aged 12–17 years. Reported prevalence increased with decreasing household educational attainment and household income but was similar regardless of whether the child had insurance coverage. Prevalence of these disorders was similar across different regions of the United States. Among the various racial and ethnic groups, the highest prevalence of behavioral or conduct disorders was found among black non-Hispanic children. National data from the 2001–2004 NHANES indicate that 2.1% of children aged 8–15 years met the criteria for conduct disorder in the past 12 months [9].

ASDs

ASDs are a group of neurodevelopmental disorders characterized by impairments in social interactions and communication as well as restricted, repetitive, and stereotyped patterns of behavior that typically emerge in the first few years of life [5] DSM-IV-TR currently classifies three ASD subtypes: 1) autistic disorder, 2) Asperger's disorder, and 3) pervasive developmental disorder not otherwise specified. [5] Studies document that children with ASDs have high levels of functional impairments and often have other developmental and mental disorders [78–80]. In addition, children with ASDs have a higher prevalence of numerous health conditions than children without ASDs, including respiratory, gastrointestinal, dermatologic, and neurologic conditions [78,80], and have a higher level of health-care services use and unmet health needs [78,80,81]. Families of children with ASDs report more parenting stress (19) and financial difficulties [13] than families of children without ASDs.

The reported prevalence of ASDs has increased markedly in recent decades, both in the United States and other industrialized countries [82–84]. In the United States, population-based ASD prevalence can be estimated using two nationally representative surveys (NHIS and NSCH) and ADDM, a monitoring network that tracks ASD prevalence in 14 population-based sites.

NHIS includes a single question on whether a doctor or other health-care provider has ever told the parent that the child has autism. The 2003 NHIS and 2003 NSCH included the same question. Because NHIS and NSCH are based on different samples and are both designed to be representative of noninstitutionalized children living in the United States, the reliability of estimates based on parent report could be assessed by comparing prevalence estimates. Results showed that autism prevalence estimates from each of the 2003 surveys were very close overall and within subgroups based on child age, sex, and race/ethnicity, suggesting high reliability [85]. Moreover, parental reports of autism were associated with expected social, emotional, and behavioral difficulties and with special health-care needs suggesting convergent validity of the autism question.

NHIS retained the same autism question through 2010. The NSCH autism question was revised after the 2003 survey; the 2007 NSCH question more explicitly asked whether a doctor or other health-care provider ever told the parent that the child has autism, Asperger's disorder, pervasive developmental disorder, or other ASD. Additionally, in the 2007 NSCH interview, parents who responded affirmatively to the first question were asked whether their child currently has autism or ASD. Thus, from NHIS data (through 2010), the prevalence can be estimated of any past autism diagnosis that might or might not have been interpreted by parents to include all ASDs. From NSCH data, the prevalence can be estimated, separately, of both any past ASD diagnosis and current report of ASD diagnosis. The ADDM estimate is based on a cumulative health and education record review of ASD diagnoses and symptoms up to age 8 years.

The 2007–2008 and 2009–2010 NHIS prevalence estimates based on parent report of autism that has ever been diagnosed for children aged 3–17 years are 0.8% and 1.1% respectively (Table 3 and Table 6). However, the difference in these estimates is primarily influenced by lower estimates for the youngest and oldest age groups in 2007–2008. Thus, on the basis of parent report, the autism prevalence among children aged 6–11 years is 1.0% according to data from the 2007–2008 NHIS and 1.1% from the 2009–2010 NHIS. The 2007 NSCH prevalence estimates for ever diagnosed ASD was 1.8% among children aged 3–17 years and 2.2% among children aged 6–11 years; both estimates are notably higher than the comparable NHIS autism estimates. Whether the higher estimates from NSCH more accurately reflect true ASD cases is difficult to assess with available data. However, the NSCH estimates of children with current autism or ASD (1.1% among children aged 3–17 years and 1.4% among children aged 6–11 years) were 40% lower than the estimates of children who ever received a diagnosis of ASD. The composite 2008 ADDM prevalence estimate for ASD among children aged 8 years was 1.1%, with a range of 0.5% to 2.1% among the 14 ADDM sites.

Estimates from these three systems show a strong predominance among boys, with boy:girl ratios ranging from 3.4 to 4.5. Other demographic differences vary somewhat among surveys and survey years. The prevalence tends to be higher among white non-Hispanic children and among children living in families in which the most highly educated adult has attained more than a high school degree. Although some regional differences exist, they are not consistent across surveys. NSCH estimates also suggest a higher prevalence among children with health insurance. Estimates did not vary by poverty level.

Mood and Anxiety Disorders

Mood and anxiety disorders represent a range of conditions commonly characterized by feelings of depression, exaggerated anxiety or fear, low self-esteem, or all of these that persist or repeat over a period of months or years [4]. Examples of mood and anxiety disorders that can be diagnosed during childhood include major depressive disorder, dysthymia, bipolar disorder, generalized anxiety, separation anxiety, posttraumatic stress disorder, obsessive-compulsive disorder, and social or specific phobias [4,86]. Mood and anxiety disorders in childhood frequently occur together [4,6,9,87] or recur over time [23,24,88]. Mood and anxiety disorders also commonly occur with other health and medical conditions, including asthma, insulin resistance, and other chronic medical conditions and might affect treatment adherence for these conditions [27,28,30,89]. Mood and anxiety disorders in children are associated with concurrent or subsequent substance use, abuse, or dependence; sexual risk-taking behaviors; criminal behavior; and poor coping and social skills [18,20,21,90–92]. Long-term effects include poor psychosocial functioning [93]; impaired functioning in domains of work, family, and parenting [94,95]; and lower educational attainment [17].

Mood Disorders (Depression)

The prevalence of depression or depressive symptoms among children in the United States is measured in several nationally representative survey systems, including NSCH, NHIS, NHANES, NSDUH, and YRBS, although the methods differ among surveys and by survey year. Estimates for other specific mood disorders (e.g., bipolar or dysthymic disorder) are not available through these survey systems. Prevalence estimates for these and other DSM-IV mental disorders among adolescents aged 13–17 years are available from NCS-A, which was administered during 2001–2004 [25,39].

The 2007 NSCH included three questions related to the presence and severity of depression among children aged 2–17 years, including whether a doctor or health-care provider had ever told the parent that their child had depression, whether the child currently had depression, and if so, whether the child's depression was mild, moderate, or severe. In 2007, NHIS used a similar question to capture the prevalence of diagnosed depression, as reported by parents, in the past 12 months among children aged 4–17 years. During 2000–2004, NHANES assessed major depression and dysthymia during the past 12 months using parent and child report using DISC-IV. Currently, NHANES uses self-reported symptoms drawn from the Patient Health Questionnaire (PHQ-9) to assess depression during the past 2 weeks among adolescents aged 12–17 years. NSDUH [96,97] uses a series of questions asked through an audio computer-assisted self-interviewing (ACASI) household interview to assess whether adolescents have experienced an MDE. MDE, as defined in NSDUH, is based on the definition of MDE in DSM-IV [5] and is measured for the lifetime and past year. Lifetime MDE is defined as having at least five or more of nine symptoms of depression in the same 2-week period in a person's lifetime, in which at least one of the symptoms was a depressed mood or loss of interest or pleasure in daily activities. Respondents who had an MDE in their lifetime were defined as having a past year MDE if they had a period of depression lasting ≥2 weeks in the past 12 months while also having some of the other symptoms of MDE. Unlike the DSM-IV criteria for MDE, no exclusions were made in NSDUH for depressive symptoms caused by medical illness, bereavement, or substance use disorders [5]. YRBS measures the prevalence of feeling sad or hopeless, which is one symptom of depression during the past 12 months, through a self-administered questionnaire completed at school by students in grades 9–12 [98].

The most recent estimates of depression among children from NSCH, NHIS, NHANES, and NSDUH are provided (Table 7). Data from the most recent NSCH based on parent report indicate that in 2007, 3.9% of children aged 3–17 years had ever received a diagnosis of depression (Table 3). As expected, this is higher than the prevalence of current depression among children aged 3–17 (2.1%), also based on parent report, in the 2007 NSCH. On the basis of data from the 2007 NHIS, the prevalence of depression based on parent report of a diagnosis in the past year among children aged 4–17 years was 3.0%.

NSDUH and NHANES collected data related to depression from adolescents aged 12–17 years. Based on self-report, the prevalence of lifetime and past year MDE among adolescents aged 12–17 years from the 2010–2011 NSDUH was 12.8% and 8.1%, respectively. The prevalence of depression in the past 2 weeks based on self-report on the PHQ-9 screener (NHANES 2007–2010) was 6.7%. According to parent report, data from the 2007 NSCH and NHIS indicate that the prevalence of diagnosed depression among adolescents aged 12–17 years was 7.1% for ever having received a diagnosis of depression, 3.5% for having current depression, and 5.1% for having had a diagnosis of depression in the past year (Table 7).

Parent-reported data from the 2007 NSCH indicate that the prevalence of depression, either current or ever diagnosed, was higher among older children (aged 12–17 years) and among children living in households with incomes

≤100% of the federal poverty level and those living in families where the most highly educated adult had attained a high school degree or less. Although the proportion of boys and girls who were reported to have ever received a diagnosis of depression or to have a current diagnosis of depression was similar, some variation was observed by age. Additional analyses of the 2007 NSCH data showed a greater proportion of girls aged 14 and 16 years had a current diagnosis of depression compared with boys (3.3% versus 2.0% and 4.3% versus 2.6%, respectively). These results are consistent with previous research that has shown varying risk for mood disorders among girls with increasing age [23,99] and also with findings from the 2010–2011 NSDUH showing a higher prevalence of MDE in the past year among adolescent girls (12.0%) than among adolescent boys (4.5%) [57]. Adolescent girls also were more likely to have a positive screen for depression (score of ≥11) through self-report on the PHQ-9 compared with adolescent boys (8.4% versus 5.2%). According to parent-report data from NSCH, the proportion of children currently or ever diagnosed with depression did not vary significantly by race or ethnicity, with the exception of non-Hispanic children of multiple races, of whom 5.9% were reported to have ever been diagnosed with depression (compared with 4.0% of white non-Hispanic children). According to the 2010–2011 NSDUH, MDE varied somewhat by race. For example, white non-Hispanic and non-Hispanic adolescents of multiple races were more likely to have had an MDE in their lifetime or in the past year than black non-Hispanic adolescents (Table 7). Differences also occurred by poverty status; adolescents living in households with incomes >100% to <200% of the federal poverty level were more likely to report MDE (both lifetime and past year) than those <100% of the federal poverty level or >200% of the federal poverty level (Table 7).

Data previously reported from the 2011 nationwide YRBS [64], which are based on student self-report, indicated that during the past year, 28.5% of high school students (most aged 14–18 years) reported that they had felt so sad or hopeless almost every day for ≥2 weeks in a row that they had stopped doing some usual activities; this finding was higher among girls (35.9%) than boys (21.5%) and higher among Hispanic students (32.6%) than white non-Hispanic (27.2%) or black non-Hispanic students (24.7%). The overall estimate of 28.5% of children reporting they so felt sad or hopeless for 2 weeks is much higher than the NSDUH lifetime or past year MDE estimates (Table 7). This might be related to numerous differences in survey methodologies, including the setting and the mode of completing YRBS (at school through a paper survey) compared with completing NSDUH (a household ACASI), as well as the fact that YRBS assesses only a single symptom of depression, whereas NSDUH assesses whether an individual meets criteria for a MDE diagnosis using DSM-IV criteria.

Anxiety Disorders

The prevalence of parent-reported anxiety among children in the United States is estimated by the 2007 NSCH and the 2007 NHIS, which focuses on phobias. No ongoing national surveillance for specific anxiety disorders (e.g., posttraumatic stress disorder or OCD) exists. Previous estimates from NCS-A might be useful for estimates of specific types of anxiety disorders in this population (Table 2); however NCS-A does not include OCD [25].

As part of the 2007 NSCH, parents or guardians of children aged 2–17 years were asked whether a doctor or health-care provider had ever told the parent that their child had anxiety problems, whether the child had current anxiety problems, and if so, whether the child's anxiety problems were mild, moderate, or severe. In 2007, NHIS used a similar question to assess the prevalence of phobias or fears diagnosed in the past 12 months as reported by parents. Parents also were asked whether their child had anxiety or stress during the past 12 months; no distinction was made between conditions identified by a health-care provider and those that were not. During 1999–2004, NHANES assessed both generalized anxiety disorder and panic disorder during the past year through self-report by children aged 8–15 years using DISC-IV.

The most recent estimates based on parent report of anxiety among children from NSCH and NHIS are provided (Table 8).

Data from the 2007 NSCH indicate that 4.7% of children aged 3–17 years had ever had anxiety, and 3% had current anxiety. The prevalence of phobias or fears diagnosed in the past year among children aged 4–17 years was 2.6%. These estimates are considerably higher than the estimates based on 2001–2004 NHANES data (using DISC-IV): 0.7% of children aged 8–15 years were reported to have generalized anxiety disorder or panic disorder in the past 12 months [9].

According to parent-reported data from NSCH, the prevalence of anxiety was higher among older children, those who had insurance coverage, and those living in households with incomes <100% of the federal poverty level (compared with those living in households with incomes >200% of the federal poverty level) regardless of whether the anxiety was current or had occurred at some point in the past. The prevalence of current anxiety was higher among boys (3.4%) than girls (2.6%). Black non-Hispanic children were less likely than white non-Hispanic children to have ever had anxiety or have current anxiety.

Substance Use Disorders and Substance Use

The use of alcohol and illicit drugs such as marijuana and inhalants among children has social, financial, and health consequences [100,101]. Substance use among adolescents can lead to poor academic performance, mental disorders, accidents and injuries, overdose, addiction, and unintended pregnancy [97,102–104]. Research indicates that early substance use initiation is associated with substance use disorders in adulthood [97]. Substance use disorders (abuse and dependence, based on DSM-IV criteria) affect approximately 20 million persons in the United States each year, including 1.7 million adolescents aged 12–17 years. Two thirds of these adolescents in 2011 had an illicit drug use disorder.

Based on NCS-A interviews conducted during 2001–2004, an estimated 8.3% of adolescents aged 13–17 years had a substance use disorder within the past year [105]. Recent findings from NSDUH indicate that the prevalence of substance use disorders among adolescents has decreased over time, from 8.9% in 2002 to 6.9% in 2011 [97]. Alcohol dependence or abuse among adolescents aged 12–17 years was 3.8% in 2011, which indicates a decline from 4.6% in 2010 and from 5.9% in 2002. The prevalence of illicit drug use disorder was higher in 2002 (5.6%) than in 2011 (4.6%). During 2004–2011, the prevalence of illicit drug use disorder has remained fairly stable (ranging from 4.3% to 4.7%).

NSDUH asks adolescents aged 12–17 years to report on symptoms of alcohol or illicit drug dependence or abuse (substance use disorder) during the past year. NSDUH defines illicit drug or alcohol dependence or abuse using criteria specified in DSM-IV [5]. Illicit drugs in NSDUH refer to marijuana/hashish, cocaine (including crack), inhalants, hallucinogens, heroin, and nonmedical use of prescription drugs.

NSDUH substance dependence questions ask about health and emotional problems associated with substance use, unsuccessful attempts to decrease use, tolerance, withdrawal, reducing other activities to use substances, spending substantial time engaging in activities related to substance use, or using the substance in greater quantities or for a longer time than intended. A respondent meets criteria for dependence when they have three or more of the symptoms of dependence. Substance abuse questions ask about problems at work, home, and school; problems with family or friends; physical danger; and legal problems because of substance use. A respondent meets criteria for abuse when they have one or more symptoms of abuse. When a respondent meets criteria for alcohol abuse or dependence or abuse of or dependence on any of the illicit drugs listed previously, they are deemed to have a substance use disorder.

NSDUH defines cigarette dependence differently from other substance use disorders. For persons who smoked cigarettes in the 30 days before the survey interview, NSDUH defines cigarette dependence using criteria derived from the Nicotine Dependence Syndrome Scale (NDSS) [106] and the Fagerstrom Test of Nicotine Dependence (FTND) [107,108]. The conceptual roots of the NDSS [106] are similar to those of the DSM-IV concept of dependence [5]. Although FTND is a multiitem measure of dependence, much of its ability to discriminate dependent smokers derives from a single item that assesses how soon after waking smokers have their first cigarette [108]. Smokers who met the criteria for either NDSS or the FTND dependence were defined as having cigarette dependence in the past month.

During 2010–2011, a total of 4.2% of adolescents were dependent on or abused alcohol in the past year (Table 9). Alcohol use disorders in the past year were higher among girls than boys and higher among non-Hispanic adolescents of multiple races, white non-Hispanic adolescents, and Hispanic adolescents than among other races; these estimates were all higher than those reported by non-Hispanic "other" adolescents and black non-Hispanic adolescents. Adolescents without health insurance were more likely to have had an alcohol use disorder in the past year compared with adolescents with health insurance. Reported estimates of alcohol use disorder were highest among adolescents living in the West. The prevalence in the West was higher than in the Midwest or the South, and the prevalence in the Northeast was higher than that in the South.

An estimated 4.7% of adolescents had an illicit drug use disorder in the past year (Table 9). The prevalence of illicit drug use disorders was similar for boys and girls. The prevalence of illicit drug use disorder in the past year was highest among non-Hispanic adolescents of multiple races and Hispanic adolescents than among white non-Hispanic adolescents, black non-Hispanic adolescents, and non-Hispanic "other" adolescents. The prevalence among non-Hispanic "other" adolescents was significantly lower than the prevalence among black non-Hispanics and white non-Hispanics. The prevalence of illicit drug use disorder was higher in the West than in other regions of the country. Estimates of illicit drug use disorder were lower among those with a family income of >200% of the federal poverty level than those with a family income that was >100% to ≤200% of the federal poverty level or ≤100% of the federal poverty level.

The specific illicit drugs used in the past month varied by age in 2011 (97). Among adolescents aged 12–13 years, 1.3% used marijuana and 1.3% used psychotherapeutic drugs (nonmedical use). Among adolescents aged 14–15 years, 6.7% used marijuana, 2.6% used psychotherapeutic drugs (nonmedical use), and 0.8% used hallucinogens.

Among adolescents aged 16–17 years, 15.1% used marijuana, 4.2% used psychotherapeutic drugs (nonmedical use), 1.6% used hallucinogens, and 0.5% used cocaine. Estimates of current use of inhalants were 1.0% for adolescents aged 12–13 years, 0.9% for adolescents aged 14–15 years, and 0.7% for adolescents aged 16–17 years.

During 2010 and 2011, a total of 2.8% of adolescents reported cigarette dependence in the past month (Table 9). Estimates of past month cigarette dependence were higher among boys than girls. Among adolescents aged 12–17 years, past month cigarette dependence was highest among non-Hispanic adolescents reporting two or more races and white non-Hispanic adolescents; these estimates were higher than among Hispanics, black non-Hispanics, and adolescents in the non-Hispanic "other" group. Adolescents without health insurance were more likely to have had past month cigarette dependence than those with health insurance. Estimates of cigarette dependence were higher in the Midwest than the South, the Northeast, and the West; the estimate in the West was lower than in the South. The percentage of adolescents with cigarette dependence in the past month was lower among those with a family income in the past year that was >200% of the federal poverty level than those with a family income >100% to ≤200% of the federal poverty level or ≤100% of the federal poverty level.

The 2010 and 2011 NSDUH indicate that 28.2% of adolescents aged 12–17 years reported using alcohol during the past year, 19.2% of adolescents used illicit drugs during the past year, and 8.1% of adolescents used cigarettes in the past month (Table 9). Past month cigarette use among girls was estimated at 7.7% and among boys was 8.4%. Data from the 2011 YRBS indicated that 38.7% of students reported using alcohol during the past month, 23.1% reported using marijuana during the past month (the most frequently used illicit drug), and 18.1% reported using cigarettes during the past month [64]. The estimates of use reported from NSDUH and YRBS might differ because of differences in methods, including different settings (NSDUH samples households and YRBS samples schools), mode, and the time period and ages assessed.

Tic Disorders (Tourette Syndrome)

Tic disorders include chronic motor or chronic vocal tic disorder, transient tic disorder, and Tourette syndrome. National surveillance data are available only for Tourette syndrome.

Tourette syndrome is characterized by the presence of persistent motor and vocal tics that last for at least a year. Tic symptoms usually begin when a child is aged 6–8 years [5]. Children with Tourette syndrome often have other mental disorders, particularly ADHD and OCD, that might contribute to the association between Tourette syndrome and lower educational outcomes, family stress, problems with social relationships, and increased health-care needs [109–111]. The only prevalence estimate of Tourette syndrome among a nationally representative sample of children was based on parent-reported data from the 2007 NSCH.

Parents were asked whether a doctor or other health-care provider had ever told them that their child had Tourette syndrome. Based on these data, 0.3% of children aged 6–17 years had ever had Tourette syndrome, as previously reported [112].

A parent-reported diagnosis of Tourette syndrome was more common in boys than girls (0.4% versus 0.2%), more likely for white non-Hispanic children (0.4%) than for Hispanic children (0.2%) or black non-Hispanic children (0.2%), and more likely for children aged 12–17 years (0.4%) than children aged 6–11 years (0.2%). Among children who had ever received a diagnosis of Tourette syndrome, 79% also had received a diagnosis of at least one other mental disorder (ADHD, behavioral problems such as conduct disorder, depression, anxiety, or an autism spectrum disorder), and 62% currently had Tourette syndrome (0.2% of children aged 6–17 years). Among those with current Tourette syndrome, most cases were described as mild (72.9%) [111].

Although the 2007 NSCH estimate relies on parent report of diagnosed Tourette syndrome, community samples that include previously undiagnosed cases report a higher prevalence of Tourette syndrome [113–115].

Indicators of Mental Health

Mentally Unhealthy Days

The mentally unhealthy days measure assesses impaired mental health using the following question: "Now thinking about your mental health, which includes stress, depression, and problems with emotions, for how many days during the past 30 days was your mental health not good?" For adolescents aged 12–17 years, NHANES is the only data source available to estimate the national prevalence of mentally unhealthy days. Higher numbers of mentally unhealthy days have been associated with higher numbers of physically unhealthy days, more activity limitations, smoking, being unable to work, lower income and education, and not having health insurance [48,49,116,117].

The mentally unhealthy days measure was dichotomized at ≥14 days or ≤13 days in the past 30 days. This level has been used previously to identify populations with more persistent mental distress and because it is similar to the timeframe used by clinicians in the assessment of the presence and severity of depression and anxiety disorders [48,118]. Based on self-reported data for the 2005–2010 data cycles, 8.3% (Table 10) of adolescents aged 12–17 years reported ≥14 mentally unhealthy days in the past month, representing nearly 2 million adolescents (Table 3). White non-Hispanic adolescents were more likely than Mexican-American adolescents to report ≥14 mentally unhealthy days.

Suicide

Suicide is defined as a death caused by self-directed injurious behavior with any intent to die as a result of the behavior [119]. Suicidal behavior is a multifaceted human behavior that is associated with psychiatric and psychological factors, biologic factors, a history of trauma, and societal and cultural factors [120]. Suicide is a problem throughout the lifespan and is the second leading cause of death among adolescents aged 12–17 years [120].

A combination of individual, relational, community, and societal factors contribute to the risk for suicide. Some of the risk factors include but are not limited to a history of mental disorders, particularly clinical depression, history of alcohol and substance abuse, barriers to accessing treatment for mental disorders, unwillingness to seek help because of the public perception attached to mental and substance abuse disorders or to suicidal thoughts, and easy access to lethal methods.

To date, protective factors have not been studied as extensively or rigorously as risk factors.

Some of the known protective factors include effective clinical treatment for mental and substance abuse disorders and physical health problems, support from ongoing medical and mental health care relationships, and family, peer, and community support [121].

Data on suicide are available from the national NVSS and NVDRS (16 states). The overall suicide rate for children aged 10–19 years was 4.5 suicides per 100,000 based on the 2010 NVSS and 4.2 suicides per 100,000 based on the 2005–2009 NVDRS (Table 11). In both data sources, the rate was higher for boys than girls and older children (aged 15–19 years) than younger children (aged 10–14 years). White non-Hispanic children and non-Hispanic children of other races had higher rates of suicide than black non-Hispanic and Hispanic children.

The most common mechanisms of injury among children were hanging/suffocation and firearms. Among children who died by suicide with known circumstances reported in NVDRS, 29.5% disclosed intent to die by suicide before the act; 35.5% had a diagnosed mental disorder at the time of death, 26.4% were under treatment for a current mental disorder at the time of death, and 21.1% had made a previous suicide attempt [11].

Nationwide estimates from the national YRBS for seriously considering suicide, making a suicide plan, and attempting suicide during the year before the 2011 YRBS have been reported [64].

The prevalence of having seriously considered attempting suicide among students was 15.8% nationwide; this was higher among girls (19.3%) than boys (12.5%) and higher among Hispanic students (16.7%) and white students (15.5%) than black students (13.2%). Nearly 13% (12.8%) of students had made a plan about how they would attempt suicide; this was higher for girls (15.0%) than boys (10.8%) and higher among Hispanic (14.3%) than white (12.1%) and black (11.1%) students. Last, 7.8% of students had attempted suicide one or more times during the year before the survey, with the prevalence of having attempted suicide being higher among girls (9.8%) than boys (5.8%) and higher among black (8.3%) and Hispanic (10.2%) than white (6.2%) students.

SAVD data indicate that a total of 28 school-associated suicides occurred among children aged 5–18 years during July 1, 2005–June 30 2011. Of the decedents in these incidents, 89% were boys, 86% were white, 11% were black, and 3% were Hispanic. The mean age and median age of the decedents was 16 years (range: 9–18 years). Most (82%) involved firearms.

Discussion

Mental disorders in children are a substantial public health concern with considerable associated costs to individuals, families, and society [6,10,15]. Although each of the surveillance systems used to collect data on mental disorders in children have different goals, each system provides a unique context; together, these systems begin to illustrate the impact of mental disorders among children.

The percentage of children reported to be experiencing these outcomes varies by condition, survey, and age. In general, ADHD was most prevalent, followed by depression, behavioral or conduct problems, anxiety, substance use disorders, ASDs, and Tourette syndrome. Because these conditions often occur together [24,26], these estimates cannot be combined for an overall estimate of the prevalence of mental disorders among children. Suicide, which often occurs in the presence of mental disorders, was the second leading cause of death among children aged 12–17 years in 2010 [11], and approximately 8% of children aged 12–17 years reported ≥14 mentally unhealthy days in the past month.

All demographic groups are affected by mental disorders in childhood, although the prevalence estimates vary by all demographic groups. The prevalence of all conditions and indicators increased with age, with the exception of ASD, which was highest in the group aged 6–11 years. Boys were more likely than girls to have most of the disorders, including ADHD, behavioral or conduct problems, ASD, anxiety, Tourette syndrome, and cigarette dependence, and boys were more likely than girls to die by suicide. Girls were more likely to have an alcohol use disorder, and adolescent girls were more likely to have depression.

The prevalences of different conditions and indicators varied by race and ethnicity. The children in the non-Hispanic multirace group generally had the highest prevalence of ADHD, depression, and substance use disorders. ADHD was lowest among Hispanic children, behavioral or conduct problems were highest among black non-Hispanic children, and ASD tended to be higher among white non-Hispanic children. Anxiety was more common among white non-Hispanic children than black non-Hispanic children. Black non-Hispanic children and non-Hispanic children of other races had a lower prevalence of alcohol use disorder.

Tourette syndrome was more common among white non-Hispanic children than black non-Hispanic children or Hispanic children.

The prevalence of ADHD, ASD, and anxiety were higher among children with health insurance, whereas those without health insurance were more likely to report substance use disorders. As household education decreased, the prevalence of parent-reported behavioral or conduct problems, depression, and anxiety increased.

As poverty levels increased, the prevalence of parent-reported ADHD, behavioral or conduct problems, depression and anxiety increased, as did illicit drug use disorders and cigarette dependence.

The prevalence of self-reported symptoms of depression (MDE, PHQ-9) was more similar among groups, with the highest prevalence in the middle income group. Regional differences generally were not consistent except that both alcohol and illicit drug use disorders were higher in the West and lower in the South, as opposed to ADHD, which was higher in the South and lower in the West.

Surveillance during 1994–2011 has identified increased reported prevalence of ADHD, ASDs, and bipolar disorder, as well as changes in patterns of drug use, among children [82–84,97,122–125]. NHIS data indicate an average annual increase in ADHD diagnosis of 3% during 1997–2006, whereas NSCH data indicate a 21.8% increase in ADHD during 2003–2007 [123,126]. NHIS data indicate a nearly fourfold increase in autism from 1997–1999 to 2006–2008; NSCH data also indicate increases in autism [82,127].

Changes in estimated prevalence over time might be associated with an actual change in prevalence, changes in case definition, changes in the public perception of mental disorders, or improvements in diagnosis, which might be associated with changes in policies and access to health care.

For example, substantive revisions have been proposed to the diagnostic criteria for many of the disorders presented in this report and will appear in the fifth edition of DSM (DSM-5), which has an expected release date of May 2013 [128–133].

Changes in the required number of symptoms, age of onset, or duration of symptoms will change the number of children with conditions that meet the case definition, which will affect prevalence. However, until these new criteria are implemented, how they will affect the prevalence rates of these disorders is unclear. Policy changes also might affect rates, including the implementation of the Mental Health Parity and Addiction Equity Act (P.L. No. 110–343) [134] and the Patient Protection and Affordable Care Act (P.L. No. 111–148) [135].

These policies promote the integration of primary and mental health services [136] and include specific provisions for children with preexisting conditions.

Additional measures or modification of existing surveillance methods that focus on children's mental health are needed to assess the potential impact of these policies.

Although numerous systems provide estimates of the prevalence of individual mental disorders in children, additional information is needed regarding the overall prevalence and impact of mental health issues on children.

First, because many of the ongoing surveillance systems discussed are based on ascertaining previously diagnosed cases, cases that have not been previously identified (e.g., those in children without access to care) are not represented in the available estimates. Second, similar to the findings of the report on surveillance of mental illness among adults [31], limited data are available on many conditions, particularly specific anxiety disorders and bipolar disorder. Third, and also similar to the adult report [31], no dedicated surveillance system on mental health in children exists. Available data do not allow for an overall estimate of the prevalence of all childhood mental disorders. Previous reports of the overall prevalence of having any mental disorder have been limited by the disorders included within the surveillance system.

The 2007 NSCH indicates that 11.3% of children aged 2–17 years had been diagnosed with an emotional, behavioral, or developmental condition [26]. Using the Composite International Diagnostic Interview to assess 14 disorders (and therefore identify previously undiagnosed cases), NCS-A found that nearly 50% of adolescents aged 13–18 years had ever had a mental disorder, including substance use disorders, with 28% meeting the criteria for severe impairment [25]. Differences in methods between these two systems, including conditions assessed, age of assessment, and how the conditions were assessed, might be responsible for the substantial difference in overall estimates.

Substantial but not insurmountable challenges to surveillance of mental disorders in children exist. An overall challenge is the establishment of consistent surveillance case definitions that allow for comparability and reliability of estimates among surveillance systems. Standard surveillance case definitions are needed to reliably categorize and count mental disorders among surveillance systems.

Criteria for mental disorders are subjective, are based on a symptom count instead of a biologic measure, might require assessment by different persons or in different settings, and might change over the course of development. In addition, there has been little study on the validation of case ascertainment methodology for surveillance of childhood mental disorders [85]. For example, although national telephone surveys are cost-effective, the validity of measuring mental disorders using the telephone needs to be studied. Even when standardized diagnostic interviews are used, the findings might differ depending on whether or not the child or parent is reporting the symptoms and might also differ with expert clinical judgment [137–140].

Different strengths and limitations are associated with surveillance efforts based on symptoms and those based on previous diagnoses. Assessing symptoms requires more time and might limit sample size but might identify previously undiagnosed cases. However, if a child is receiving adequate treatment for a condition, symptoms might not be reported, and the case might be missed. Relying on report of previous diagnoses takes little time and can be easily integrated into ongoing surveys but does not catch undiagnosed cases and might include misdiagnosed cases.

To improve comprehensive surveillance of mental disorders among children, validation of current methods (e.g., studies comparing parent report or screening instruments with diagnostic interviews) is needed, including those that can be incorporated into national surveys. In addition, targeted and longitudinal epidemiologic studies are needed to complement national surveys to better describe mental disorders among children, as well as their impact and course during development. For example, ADDM data address issues regarding ASDs, whereas NCS-A provides national estimates for a large number of mental disorders based on a clinical interview.

The Great Smoky Mountains Study and the Project to Learn about ADHD in Youth (PLAY) monitored community samples of children longitudinally [23,141].

Longitudinal studies can provide data on incidence, emerging health risk behaviors and comorbid conditions, and risk and protective factors to guide intervention strategies for diagnosis, treatment, and prevention. Targeted epidemiologic studies also can increase understanding of mental disorders that are difficult to diagnose and are not being monitored in existing surveillance systems, including childhood-onset schizophrenia [142]; however, they might not be generalizable to the U.S. population.

Validation and complementary approaches to better document the prevalence and impact of childhood mental disorders might best be achieved by strengthening partnerships and strategic coordination of surveillance efforts. One way this has been addressed is through the partnership between HRSA and CDC in the sponsorship and execution of NSCH and its associated survey, the National Survey of Children with Special Health Care Needs. In addition, SAMHSA, NIMH, and CDC are working together to develop an indicator of serious emotional disturbance [143].

CDC collaborated with several organizations including NIMH and the Department of Veterans Affairs, state health departments, and clinicians over several years to develop uniform definitions and recommended data elements for surveillance of self-directed violence [119]. NIMH, HRSA, and CDC collaborated on the Survey of Pathways to Diagnosis and Services, a follow-back survey with parents of children with ASD, intellectual disability, or developmental delay (or all of these) when first interviewed for the 2009–2010 National Survey of Children with Special Health Care Needs. This survey examined the emergence of symptoms; the history of diagnoses, treatments, and interventions used; and current behavioral, diagnostic, and functional status. Collaboration among partnering agencies could improve surveillance efforts.

Although this report focused on selected mental disorders and indicators of mental health among children, surveillance of mental health service use [144] and use of psychotropic medications also are important for understanding the public health impact of mental disorders among children [145–149].

In addition, more attention to the prevalence and treatment of mental disorders among preschool-age children is needed [146,149].

Surveillance is a critical first step in the public health approach to mental health among children.

Data collection and monitoring are important to identify need and target resources at the national, state, and local levels. Surveillance data can help prioritize areas for research on risk and protective factors and provide empirical evidence to develop effective interventions that can prevent mental disorders and promote mental health as recommended by a recent IOM report [6,37,150].

As intervention and prevention strategies are implemented, surveillance is needed to continually monitor progress in reducing the impact of mental disorders and improving mental health.

Table 1. Federal surveys and surveillance systems that collect data on mental disorders among children

Name, website, and sponsor	Description	Method of data collection	Survey topics related to children	Mental health topics and questions related to children	Populations and periodicity
National Survey of Children's Health (NSCH) http://www.cdc.gov/nchs/slaits/nsch.htm Sponsor: Health Resources and Services Administration Administrator: CDC National Center for Health Statistics	NSCH examines the physical and emotional health of children aged 0–17 years, emphasizing factors that might relate to the well-being of children.	Telephone interviews, with National Immunization Survey sampling frame	Physical, emotional, and dental health Medical home Child, family, and neighborhood well-being Children with special health-care needs Health-care access, use, and barriers Satisfaction with health-care services Neighborhood and community characteristics, including perceived safety, violence, and social capital Health insurance	Activity, social, or learning limitation resulting from mental, emotional, or behavior problems Common acute and chronic conditions (including learning disability, ADHD, depression, anxiety, behavior and conduct disorders, ASD, Tourette syndrome, and epilepsy) Sleep and exercise difficulties Social behavior, emotional difficulties, and school engagement Mental health-care treatment and services used	Representative sample nationally and within each state of households with children Approximately 95,000 childrenaged ≤17 years Periodic: data collected approximately every 4 years and currently available for 2003, 2007, and 2011–2012
National Survey on Drug Use and Health (NSDUH) http://www.samhsa.gov/data/NSDUH.aspx Sponsor: Substance Abuse and Mental Health Services Administration	NSDUH data are used to provide national and state-level estimates on the use of tobacco products, alcohol, illicit drugs (including nonmedical use of prescription drugs), and mental illness in the United States.	In-person household interviews	Timing and frequency of use of tobacco products, alcohol, marijuana, cocaine, heroin, inhalants, hallucinogens, and prescription drugs (nonmedical use) Risk and protective factors Employment, income,	Lifetime and past year major depressive episode Substance use disorder and treatment Level of impairment resulting from major depressive disorder, substance use, and substance use disorder Treatment for depression Mental health service use	State and nationally representative sample 7,200 primary sampling units each year and approximately 70,000 respondents aged ≥12 years, including 23,000 aged 12–17 years

Name, website, and sponsor	Description	Method of data collection	Survey topics related to children	Mental health topics and questions related to children	Populations and periodicity
			program participation, health insurance, and education Health conditions Health-care use	Parental mental illness, substance use, and substance use disorder	and 23,000 aged 18–25 years Annual and continuous since 1992
National Violent Death Reporting System (NVDRS) http://www.cdc.gov/ncipc/wisqars/NVDRS/About-NVDRS.htm#disclaimer Sponsor: CDC National Center for Injury Prevention and Control	NVDRS is a state-based surveillance system that links data from law enforcement, coroners and medical examiners, vital statistics, and crime laboratories to assist participating states in designing and implementing tailored prevention and intervention efforts. An incident-based, relational database collects and stores the data and is available free of charge from the NVDRS Web-	State-collected information from numerous data sources, including death certificates, coroner and medical examiner records, police records, and input from data abstractors	*Violent deaths:* Suicides Homicides Deaths from legal intervention (a subtype of homicide) Child maltreatment deaths Intimate partner homicides *Other deaths:* Deaths from undetermined intent Unintentional firearm deaths	Intent, cause, and manner of injury (including suicide and homicide) Child maltreatment Poisoning (alcohol or other drug) Type of victim-suspect relationship *Suicide and undetermined death circumstances:* Current depressed mood	19 states; not nationally representative All ages Annual since 2003
	based Injury Statistics Query and Reporting System (WISQARS).			Current treatment for mental health problem Ever treated for mental health problem Suicide note Disclosure of intent to commit suicide History of suicide attempts Crisis in past 2 weeks Intimate partner problem Other relationship problem	

Table 1. (Continued)

Name, website, and sponsor	Description	Method of data collection	Survey topics related to children	Mental health topics and questions related to children	Populations and periodicity
				Alcohol dependence Other substance problem	
National Vital Statistics System (NVSS) http://www.cdc.gov/nchs/deaths Source: CDC National Center for Health Statistics	NVSS mortality data provide demographic, geographic, and cause-of-death information about persons who have died in the United States in a given year.	Compilation of data from all death certificates filed in the United States into an annual file	Underlying cause of death Multiple causes of death Year, month, and day of week of death Place of death Residence of decedent (state, county, city, population size, standard metropolitan statistical area, and metropolitan and nonmetropolitan counties) State and county of occurrence Demographic information about decedent (e.g., age at death, education, Hispanic origin, marital status, race, sex, state of birth)	Information for children who die as a result of homicide, suicide, or other external causes of death (e.g., drug overdose) Underlying cause of death Multiple causes of death	National (including all states and DC, with available data on Puerto Rico, the U.S. VirginIslands, Guam, American Samoa, and the Northern Mariana Islands) All ages Annual since 1960

Name, website, and sponsor	Description	Method of data collection	Survey topics related to children	Mental health topics and questions related to children	Populations and periodicity
National Youth Risk Behavior Survey (YRBS) http://www.cdc.gov/yrbs Sponsor: CDC National Center for HIV/AIDS, Viral Hepatitis, STD, and TB Prevention	The national YRBS is a survey that is part of a large surveillance system, the Youth Risk Behavior Surveillance System, which also includes state and local school-based surveys. The national YRBS monitors priority health-risk behaviors that contribute substantially to the leading causes of death, disability, and social problems among U.S. children and adults.	School-based survey	Tobacco use Dietary behaviors Inadequate physical activity Alcohol and other drug use Sexual behaviors that contribute to unintended pregnancy and sexually transmitted diseases Behaviors that might contribute to unintentional injuries and violence	Activity limitations resulting from mental or emotional problems Suicide ideation and attempt behaviors Alcohol, tobacco, and other drug use Drug use during sexual activity	Nationally representative 16,000 public and private high school students (grades 9—12), with available state and local data Oversample of blacks and Hispanics Biennial since 1991 (odd years)
School-Associated Violent Death Study (SAVD)	SAVD is an ongoing, national study that monitors trends related to school-associated violent deaths	Compiled data from media databases (such as Lexis-Nexis), law enforcement officials,	Common features of the event Potential risk factors for perpetration and	At the time of the event: Demonstration of symptoms consistent	National Only includes violent deaths associated with U.S.
http://www.cdc.gov/violenceprevention/youthviolence/schoolviolence/SAVD.html Sponsors: CDC National Center for Injury Prevention and Control, the Department of Education, and the Department of Justice	(including suicide), identifying risk factors, and assessing the effects of prevention efforts.	and school officials, mortality data from the National Center for Health Statistics, and data from the U.S. Department of Education	victimization Possible prevention measures Warning signs Risk estimates	with ADHD or another hyperactivity disorder Diagnosis of ADHD or another hyperactivity disorder Treatment of ADHD or another hyperactivity disorder Presence of a diagnosed learning disability Year before the event: Receipt of school-sponsored	elementary and secondary schools, both public and private All ages Annual since 1992

Table 1. (Continued)

Name, website, and sponsor	Description	Method of data collection	Survey topics related to children	Mental health topics and questions related to children	Populations and periodicity
				psychological counseling services Treatment for depression Presence of thoughts or threats of suicide Previous suicide attempts	

Abbreviations: ADHD = attention-deficit/hyperactivity disorder; ASD = autism spectrum disorder; IQ = intelligence quotient; PHQ-9 = nine-item Patient Health Questionnaire.

Table 2. Prevalence estimates of childhood mental disorders for which data are not routinely collected

Disorder	Surveillance system	Estimate (%)
Anxiety disorders		
Agoraphobia	NCS-A*	2.4
Generalized anxiety disorder	NCS-A* NHANES†	2.2 0.3
Obsessive-compulsive disorder	DSM-IV§	1.0–2.3
Panic disorder	NCS-A* NHANES†	2.3 0.4
Posttraumatic stress disorder	NCS-A*	5.0
Separation anxiety	NCS-A*	7.6
Social phobia	NCS-A*	9.1
Specific phobia	NCS-A*	19.3

Disorder	Surveillance system	Estimate (%)
Bipolar I or II disorder	NCS-A*	2.9
Childhood onset schizophrenia	Primary study¶	0.014
Eating disorder	NHANES†	0.1

Abbreviations: DISC = Diagnostic Interview Schedule for Children; DSM-IV = Diagnostic and Statistical Manual of Mental Disorders, 4th edition, text revision; NCS-A: National Comorbidity Survey—Adolescent Supplement; NHANES = National Health and Nutrition Examination Survey.

* NCS-A 2001–2004, adolescents aged 13–18 years, lifetime prevalence. (Source: Merikangas KR, He JP, Burstein M, et al. Lifetime prevalence of mental disorders in U.S. adolescents: results from the National Comorbidity Survey Replication— Adolescent Supplement [NCS-A]. J Am Acad Child Adolesc Psychiatry 2010;49:980–9.)

† NHANES 2001–2004, children aged 8–15 years, 12-month estimate based on DISC. (Source: Merikangas KR, He JP, Brody D, Fisher PW, Bourdon K, Koretz DS. Prevalence and treatment of mental disorders among U.S. children in the 2001–2004 NHANES. Pediatrics 2010;125:75–81.)

§ The estimates for obsessive-compulsive disorder were taken from DSM-IV because no national estimates were identified; the estimate is for lifetime for children and adolescents. (Source: American Psychiatric Association. Diagnostic and statistical manual of mental disorders. 4th ed, text revision. Washington, DC: American Psychiatric Association; 2000.)

¶ Childhood-onset schizophrenia is defined as onset before age 13 years. Child-onset schizophrenia is not included in ongoing national surveillance, at least in part because of its rarity and the challenges in accurately identifying schizophrenia through survey measures or nonclinical interviews. (Sources: Thomsen PH. Schizophrenia with childhood and adolescent onset—a nationwide register-based study. Acta Psychiatr Scand 1996;94:187–93; Gochman P, Miller R, Rapoport JL. Childhood-onset schizophrenia: the challenge of diagnosis. Curr Psychiatry Rep 2011;13:321–2; and McKenna K, Gordon CT, Rapoport JL. Childhood-onset schizophrenia: timely neurobiological research. J Am Acad Child Adolesc Psychiatry 1994; 33:771–81.)

Table 3. Estimated prevalence and number of children with mental disorders, by surveillance system, age range, and year — National Health Interview Survey, National Survey of Children's Health, National Survey on Drug Use and Health, and National Health and Nutrition Examination Survey, United States, 2007–2011

Condition	Surveillance system and years	Age range (yrs)	Sample size (no. of persons surveyed)	Weighted prevalence (%)	Weighted* no. of children
Attention-deficit/hyperactivity	NHIS 2007–2008	3–17	14,970	7.6 (ever)	4,718,000
disorder	NHIS 2009–2010	3–17	18,411	8.5 (ever)	5,232,000
	NHIS 2011	3–17	10,554	8.4 (ever)	5,246,000
	NSCH 2007	3–17	78,042	8.9 (ever)	5,482,000
	NSCH 2007	3–17	78,042	6.8 (current)	4,188,000
Behavioral or conduct problems	NSCH 2007	3–17	78,042	4.6 (ever)	2,833,000
	NSCH 2007	3–17	78,042	3.5 (current)	2,156,000
Autism spectrum disorders	NHIS 2007–2008	3–17	14,970	0.8 (ever autism)	485,000
	NHIS 2009–2010	3–17	18,411	1.1 (ever autism)	667,000
	NSCH 2007	3–17	78,042	1.8 (ever ASD)	1,109,000
	NSCH 2007	3–17	78,042	1.1 (current ASD)	678,000
Depression	NHIS 2007	4–17	7,103	3.0 (past year)	1,706,000
	NSCH 2007	3–17	78,042	3.9 (ever)	2,402,000
	NSCH 2007	3–17	78,042	2.1 (current)	1,293,000
	NSDUH 2010–2011	12–17	45,500	12.8 (lifetime)	3,106,000
	NSDUH 2010–2011	12–17	45,500	8.1 (MDE past year)	1,961,000
	NHANES 2007–2010	12–17	1,782	6.7 (PHQ-9, past 2 weeks)	1,708,000
Anxiety	NHIS 2007	4–17	7,103	2.6 (phobia, past year)	1,515,000
	NSCH 2007	3–17	78,042	4.7 (ever)	2,895,000
	NSCH 2007	3–17	78,042	3.0 (current)	1,848,000
Alcohol use disorder	NSDUH 2010–2011	12–17	45,500	4.2 (past year)	1,028,000
Illicit drug use disorder	NSDUH 2010–2011	12–17	45,500	4.7 (past year)	1,155,000
Cigarette dependence	NSDUH 2010–2011	12–17	45,500	2.8 (past month)	691,000

Condition	Surveillance system and years	Age range (yrs)	Sample size (no. of persons surveyed)	Weighted prevalence (%)	Weighted* no. of children
Tourette syndrome	NSCH 2007	6–17	64,034	0.3 (ever)	148,000
			64,034	0.2 (current)	99,000
≥14 mentally unhealthy days	NHANES 2005–2010	12–17	3,312	8.3 (past 30 days)	1,995,000

Abbreviations: MDE = major depressive episode; NHANES = National Health and Nutrition Examination Survey; NHIS = National Health Interview Survey; NSCH = National Survey of Children's Health; NSDUH = National Survey on Drug Use and Health; PHQ-9 = nine-item Patient Health Questionnaire.

* Weighted estimates of the number of children with mental disorders or with ≥14 mentally unhealthy days were calculated by multiplying the prevalence estimate by the U.S. Census Bureau's population estimate of the total number of noninstitutionalized children in the age group, as determined by census population estimates for the year of the survey.

Table 4. Prevalence of children aged 3–17 years who ever received a diagnosis of ADHD or with current ADHD, by sociodemographic characteristics and year — National Health Interview Survey and National Survey of Children's Health, United States, 2007–2011

Characteristic	Ever received a diagnosis of ADHD (parent report)								Current ADHD (parent report)	
	NHIS 2007–2008 (N = 14,970 persons surveyed)		NHIS 2009–2010 (N = 18,411 persons surveyed)		NHIS 2011 (N = 10,554 persons surveyed)		NSCH 2007 (N = 78,042 persons surveyed)		NSCH 2007 (N = 78,042 personssurveyed)	
	%	(95% CI)	%	(95% CI)	%	(95% CI)	%	(95% CI)	%	(95% CI)
Sex										
Male	10.6	(9.7–11.4)	11.5	(10.7–12.3)	12.0	(11.0–13.1)	12.3	(11.6–13.1)	9.6	(8.9–10.4)
Female	4.6	(4.0–5.3)	5.4	(4.8–6.0)	4.7	(4.0–5.6)	5.3	(4.8–5.9)	3.8	(3.4–4.2)
Age group (yrs)										
3–5	2.1	(1.5–2.8)	2.5	(1.9–3.4)	2.1	(1.4–3.0)	1.5	(1.1–1.9)	1.1	(0.9–1.5)
6–11	7.4	(6.6–8.3)	8.2	(7.4–9.0)	8.4	(7.4–9.5)	9.1	(8.3–9.9)	7.5	(6.8–8.2)
12–17	10.8	(9.8–11.8)	11.9	(11.0–12.9)	11.9	(10.7–13.2)	12.4	(11.5–13.3)	8.8	(8.1–9.6)

Table 4. (Continued)

Characteristic	Ever received a diagnosis of ADHD (parent report)								Current ADHD (parent report)	
	NHIS 2007–2008 (N = 14,970 persons surveyed)		NHIS 2009–2010 (N = 18,411 persons surveyed)		NHIS 2011 (N = 10,554 persons surveyed)		NSCH 2007 (N = 78,042 persons surveyed)		NSCH 2007 (N = 78,042 personssurveyed)	
	%	(95% CI)	%	(95% CI)	%	(95% CI)	%	(95% CI)	%	(95% CI)
Race/Ethnicity*										
Hispanic	4.1	(3.4–4.9)	4.6	(3.9–5.4)	5.6	(4.6–6.8)	5.4	(4.4–6.6)	4.0	(3.1–5.0)
Black, non-Hispanic	8.1	(6.9–9.5)	10.3	(9.1–11.7)	8.8	(7.3–10.5)	10.0	(8.8–11.4)	7.7	(6.6–9.0)
White, non-Hispanic	9.1	(8.3–10.0)	10.0	(9.2–10.8)	10.1	(9.1–11.2)	10.0	(9.4–10.6)	7.6	(7.0–8.1)
Multirace, non-Hispanic	10.2	(7.3–14.0)	11.5	(8.6–15.2)	5.5	(3.4–8.6)	13.0	(10.4–16.2)	10.2	(7.9–13.0)
Other, non-Hispanic	3.1	(1.8–5.3)	2.0	(1.4–2.9)	4.1	(2.4–6.9)	4.0	(3.1–5.1)	3.0	(2.2–3.9)
Highest education in household†										
Less than high school	6.5	(4.9–8.5)	7.9	(6.5–9.5)	7.7	(6.1–9.7)	8.5	(7.1–10.2)	6.6	(5.3–8.1)
High school graduate	8.9	(7.8–10.1)	10.5	(9.3–11.7)	7.5	(6.3–9.0)	11.8	(10.5–13.2)	8.7	(7.7–9.8)
More than high school	7.4	(6.8–8.2)	8.0	(7.4–8.7)	8.8	(8.0–9.7)	8.1	(7.6–8.7)	6.3	(5.8–6.8)
Insurance										
Yes	7.9	(7.3–8.5)	8.7	(8.2–9.3)	8.7	(8.0–9.5)	9.2	(8.7–9.7)	7.1	(6.7–7.6)
No	5.4	(4.2–6.9)	5.9	(4.6–7.5)	4.7	(3.2–6.7)	6.3	(4.9–8.2)	3.5	(2.7–4.5)
Region										
Northeast	6.8	(5.8–8.0)	8.6	(7.4–9.9)	7.5	(6.0–9.4)	8.8	(7.8–9.9)	7.0	(6.1–8.0)
Midwest	8.8	(7.5–10.2)	9.4	(8.3–10.7)	8.7	(7.3–10.3)	9.3	(8.6–10.1)	7.1	(6.5–7.8)
South	8.9	(8.0–10.0)	10.1	(9.2–11.0)	10.3	(9.2–11.6)	10.3	(9.5–11.1)	7.7	(7.1–8.5)

Characteristic	Ever received a diagnosis of ADHD (parent report)								Current ADHD (parent report)	
	NHIS 2007–2008 (N = 14,970 persons surveyed)		NHIS 2009–2010 (N = 18,411 persons surveyed)		NHIS 2011 (N = 10,554 persons surveyed)		NSCH 2007 (N = 78,042 persons surveyed)		NSCH 2007 (N = 78,042 personssurveyed)	
	%	(95% CI)	%	(95% CI)	%	(95% CI)	%	(95% CI)	%	(95% CI)
West	5.1	(4.3–6.0)	5.2	(4.4–6.1)	6.0	(4.9–7.3)	6.6	(5.4–7.9)	4.8	(3.9–6.0)
Poverty-income ratio§										
≤100% FPL	8.9	(7.5–10.4)	11.4	(10.1–12.7)	10.5	(8.9–12.4)	11.1	(9.9–12.4)	8.7	(7.7–10.0)
>100% to ≤200% FPL	8.6	(7.3–10.0)	9.2	(8.0–10.6)	6.7	(5.6–8.1)	9.7	98.6–11.0)	7.2	(6.3–8.3)
>200% FPL	6.9	(6.3–7.6)	7.1	(6.5–7.8)	8.3	(7.5–9.3)	8.0	(7.5–8.6)	6.1	(5.6–6.6)
Total	7.6	(7.1–8.2)	8.5	(8.0–9.0)	8.4	(7.8–9.1)	8.9	(8.4–9.4)	6.8	(6.4–7.2)

Abbreviations: ADHD = attention-deficit/hyperactivity disorder; CI = confidence interval; FPL = federal poverty level; NHIS = National Health Interview Survey; NSCH = National Survey of Children's Health.

* Other, non-Hispanic, includes American Indian/Alaska Native, Hawaiian/other Pacific Islander, and Asian. Persons categorized as multirace selected more than one race. † The highest education in the household is based on the highest education of adults in the sample child's family for NHIS and on the education of parents or respondents (adults) for NSCH.

§ FPL is based on family income and family size and composition using federal poverty thresholds that are updated annually by the U.S. Census Bureau using the change in the average annual consumer price index for all urban consumers. (Additional information available at http://www.census.gov/hhes/www/poverty/index.html.)

Table 5. Prevalence of children aged 3–17 years who ever received a diagnosis of behavioral or conduct problems or with current behavioral or conduct problems, by sociodemographic characteristics — National Survey of Children's Health, United States, 2007

Characteristic	Ever received a diagnosis of behavioral or conduct problems (parent report) (N = 78,042 persons surveyed)		Current behavioral or conduct problems (parent report) (N = 78,042 persons surveyed)	
	%	(95% CI)	%	(95% CI)

Table 5. (Continued)

Characteristic	Ever received a diagnosis of behavioral or conduct problems (parent report) (N = 78,042 persons surveyed)		Current behavioral or conduct problems (parent report) (N = 78,042 persons surveyed)	
	%	(95% CI)	%	(95% CI)
Sex				
Male	6.2	(5.7–6.8)	4.6	(4.1–5.1)
Female	3.0	(2.6–3.4)	2.2	(1.9–2.7)
Age group (yrs)				
3–5	1.5	(1.2–1.8)	1.3	(1.0–1.6)
6–11	5.1	(4.5–5.8)	3.8	(3.3–4.4)
12–17	5.7	(5.2–6.3)	4.2	(3.7–4.7)
Race/Ethnicity*				
Hispanic	3.9	(3.1–5.0)	3.2	(2.4–4.2)
Black, non-Hispanic	8.1	(6.9–9.4)	6.0	(5.0–7.2)
White, non-Hispanic	4.2	(3.7–4.6)	3.0	(2.7–3.4)
Multirace, non-Hispanic	4.8	(3.6–6.2)	4.0	(2.9–5.4)
Other, non-Hispanic	2.6	(1.8–3.7)	1.6	(1.0–2.6)
Highest education in household†				
Less than high school	7.3	(5.8–9.0)	6.1	(4.8–7.7)
High school graduate	7.0	(6.1–8.1)	5.3	(4.5–6.3)
More than high school	3.5	(3.2–3.9)	2.5	(2.2–2.9)

Characteristic	Ever received a diagnosis of behavioral or conduct problems (parent report) (N = 78,042 persons surveyed)		Current behavioral or conduct problems (parent report) (N = 78,042 persons surveyed)	
	%	(95% CI)	%	(95% CI)
Insurance				
Yes	4.7	(4.3– 5.1)	3.5	(3.2–3.8)
No	4.0	(2.8– 5.8)	3.3	(2.2–5.1)
Region Northeast	5.1	(4.3–6.1)	3.7	(2.9–4.6)
Midwest	4.6	(4.1–5.2)	3.3	(2.9–3.8)
South	5.2	(4.6–5.9)	4.0	(3.5–4.6)
West	3.4	(2.7–4.3)	2.6	(2.0–3.5)
Poverty-income ratio§				
≤100% FPL	9.0	(7.9–10.3)	7.3	(6.3–8.4)
>100% to ≤200% FPL	5.9	(5.0–6.9)	4.5	(3.7–5.4)
>200% FPL	2.9	(2.6–3.3)	2.0	(1.7–2.3)
Total	4.6	(4.3–5.0)	3.5	(3.1–3.8)

Abbreviations: CI = confidence interval; FPL = federal poverty level.

* Other, non-Hispanic, includes American Indian/Alaska Native, Hawaiian/other Pacific Islander, and Asian. Persons categorized as multirace selected more than one race.

† The highest education in the household is based on the education of parents or respondents (adults).

§ FPL is based on family income and family size and composition using federal poverty thresholds that are updated annually by the U.S. Census Bureau using the change in the average annual consumer price index for all urban consumers. (Additional information available at http://www. census.gov/hhes/www/poverty/index.html.)

Table 6. Prevalence of children who ever received a diagnosis of autism or autism spectrum disorder or with current autism or autism spectrum disorder, by sociodemographic characteristics and year — National Health Interview Survey, National Survey of Children's Health, and the Autism and Developmental Disabilities Monitoring Network, United States, 2007–2010

	Ever received a diagnosis of autism or ASD (parent report)*						Current autism or ASD (parent report)*		Met surveillance case definition at time of interview (health and educationrecord reviews)	
	NHIS 2007–2008 Ages: 3–17 years (N = 14,970 persons surveyed)		NHIS 2009–2010 Ages: 3–17 years (N = 18,411 persons surveyed)		NSCH 2007 Ages: 3–17 years (N = 78,042 persons surveyed)		NSCH 2007 Ages: 3–17 years (N = 78,042 persons surveyed)		ADDM 2008 ASD age: 8 years† (N = 337,093 persons surveyed)	
Characteristic	%	(95% CI)	%	(95% CI)	%	(95% CI)	%	(95% CI)	%	(95% CI)
Sex										
Male	1.3	(1.0–1.6)	1.7	(1.4–2.0)	2.8	(2.4–3.3)	1.7	(1.4–2.1)	1.8	(1.8–1.9)
Female	0.3	(0.2–0.4)	0.5	(0.3–0.7)	0.8	(0.6–1.0)	0.4	(0.3–0.6)	0.4	(0.37–0.43)
Age group (yrs) 3–5	0.8	(0.5–1.2)	1.1	(0.8–1.6)	1.6	(1.2–2.3)	0.9	(0.6–1.2)	NA	NA
6–11	1.0	(0.7–1.3)	1.1	(0.8–1.4)	2.2	(1.8–2.7)	1.4	(1.1–1.7)	NA	NA
12–17	0.6	(0.4–0.9)	1.1	(0.8–1.4)	1.6	(1.3–1.9)	1.0	(0.8–1.2)	NA	NA
Race/Ethnicity§										
Hispanic	0.5	(0.3–0.9)	0.7	(0.5–1.0)	1.3	(0.9–2.0)	1.0	(0.6–1.7)	0.8	(0.7–0.9)
Black, non-Hispanic	0.4¶	(0.2–0.8)¶	0.9	(0.5–1.4)	1.9	(1.3–2.8)	0.6	(0.4–1.0)	1.0	(1.0–1.1)
White, non-Hispanic	0.9	(0.7–1.2)	1.3	(1.0–1.6)	2.0	(1.7–2.3)	1.3	(1.1–1.5)	1.2	(1.2–1.3)

	Ever received a diagnosis of autism or ASD (parent report)*						Current autism or ASD (parent report)*		Met surveillance case definition at time of interview (health and educationrecord reviews)	
	NHIS 2007–2008 Ages: 3–17 years (N = 14,970 persons surveyed)		NHIS 2009–2010 Ages: 3–17 years (N = 18,411 persons surveyed)		NSCH 2007 Ages: 3–17 years (N = 78,042 persons surveyed)		NSCH 2007 Ages: 3–17 years (N = 78,042 persons surveyed)		ADDM 2008 ASD age: 8 years† (N = 337,093 persons surveyed)	
Characteristic	%	(95% CI)	%	(95% CI)	%	(95% CI)	%	(95% CI)	%	(95% CI)
Multirace, non-Hispanic	—**	—	2.0¶	(1.1–3.9)¶	1.1	(0.8–1.6)	0.7	(0.4–1.1)	NA	
Other, non-Hispanic	1.1¶	(0.4–2.6)¶	0.7¶	(0.4–1.5)¶	1.8	(1.0–3.4)	0.7	(0.4–1.2)	1.0	(0.8–1.2)
Highest education in household††										
Less than high school	0.3¶	(0.1–0.6)¶	0.5¶	(0.2–1.0)¶	2.6	(1.6–4.0)	1.7	(1.0–3.0)	NA	NA
High school graduate	0.6	(0.4–0.9)	0.8	(0.5–1.3)	1.8	(1.4–2.4)	0.7	(0.5–0.9)	NA	NA
More than high school	0.9	(0.7–1.2)	1.2	(1.0–1.5)	1.8	(1.5–2.0)	1.2	(1.0–1.4)	NA	NA
Insurance										
Yes	0.8	(0.7–1.0)	1.1	(0.9–1.3)	1.9	(1.7–2.2)	1.2	(1.0–1.4)	NA	NA
No	—	—	—	—	1.0	(0.6–1.7)	0.5	(0.3–0.8)	NA	NA
Region Northeast	0.8	(0.5–1.4)	1.3	(0.9–1.9)	2.3	(1.8–3.0)	1.3	(1.0–1.8)	NA	NA
Midwest	1.0	(0.7–1.3)	1.4	(1.0–2.0)	1.8	(1.6–2.2)	1.2	(1.0–1.5)	NA	NA
South	0.7	(0.5–1.0)	0.8	(0.6–1.1)	1.8	(1.4–2.3)	1.1	(0.8–1.5)	NA	NA
West	0.7	(0.4–1.2)	1.0	(0.7–1.4)	1.5	(1.0–2.1)	0.8	(0.6–1.2)	NA	NA
Poverty-income ratio§§										
≤100% FPL	0.9	(0.5–1.6)	1.1	(0.7–1.6)	1.9	(1.4–2.7)	1.1	(0.7–1.7)	NA	NA
>100% to ≤200% FPL	0.6	(0.3–0.9)	1.0	(0.7–1.6)	1.9	(1.4–2.5)	1.0	(0.7–1.3)	NA	NA

Table 6. (Continued)

	Ever received a diagnosis of autism or ASD (parent report)*						Current autism or ASD (parent report)*		Met surveillance case definition at time of interview (health and educationrecord reviews)	
	NHIS 2007–2008 Ages: 3–17 years (N = 14,970 persons surveyed)		NHIS 2009–2010 Ages: 3–17 years (N = 18,411 persons surveyed)		NSCH 2007 Ages: 3–17 years (N = 78,042 persons surveyed)		NSCH 2007 Ages: 3–17 years (N = 78,042 persons surveyed)		ADDM 2008 ASD age: 8 years† (N = 337,093 persons surveyed)	
Characteristic	%	(95% CI)	%	(95% CI)	%	(95% CI)	%	(95% CI)	%	(95% CI)
>200% FPL	0.8	(0.6–1.1)	1.1	(0.9–1.4)	1.8	(1.5–2.1)	1.2	(0.9–1.4)	NA	NA
Total	0.8	(0.6–1.0)	1.1	(0.9–1.3)	1.8	(1.6–2.1)	1.1	(0.9–1.3)	1.1	(1.1–1.2)

Abbreviations: ADDM = Autism and Developmental Disabilities and Monitoring Network; ASD = autism spectrum disorder; CI = confidence interval; FPL = federal poverty level; NA = not available; NHIS = National Health Interview Survey; NSCH = National Survey of Children's Health.

* Autism was addressed by NHIS; ASD was addressed by NSCH.

† ADDM data based on 14 population-based sites.

§ Other, non-Hispanic, includes American Indian/Alaska Native, Hawaiian/other Pacific Islander, and Asian. Persons categorized as multirace selected more than one race.

¶ Relative standard error is >30% and <50%.

** Data suppressed because relative standard error is ≥50%.

†† The highest education in the household is based on the highest education of adults in the sample child's family for NHIS and on the education of parents or respondents (adults) for NSCH.

§§ FPL is based on family income and family size and composition using federal poverty thresholds that are updated annually by the U.S. Census Bureau using the change in the average annual consumer price index for all urban consumers. (Additional information available at http://www.census.gov/hhes/www/poverty/index.html.)

Table 7. Prevalence of children who, during the past 12 months, received a diagnosis of depression or had a major depressive episode; who ever received a diagnosis of depression or had a major depressive episode; and with current depression or depression within the past 2 weeks, by sociodemographic characteristics and year — National Health Interview Survey, National Survey of Children's Health, National Survey on Drug Use and Health, and National Health and Nutrition Examination Survey, United States, 2007–2011

Received a diagnosis of depression during past 12 months (parent report)			Ever received a diagnosis of depression (parent report)		Current depression (parent report)		Lifetime major depressive episode (child report)		Major depressive episode during past 12 months (child report)		Current depression during past 2 weeks (child report, score of ≥10 on PHQ-9)	
	NHIS 2007 Ages: 4–17 years (N = 7,103 persons surveyed)		NSCH 2007 Ages: 3–17 years (N = 78,042 persons surveyed)		NSCH 2007 Ages: 3–17 years (N = 78,042 persons surveyed)		NSDUH 2010–2011 Ages: 12–17 years (N = 45,500 persons surveyed)*		NSDUH 2010–2011 Ages: 12–17 years (N = 45,500 persons surveyed)*		NHANES 2007–2010 Ages: 12–17 years (N = 1,782 persons surveyed)	
Characteristic	%	(95% CI)	%	(95% CI)	%	(95% CI)	%	(95% CI)	%	(95% CI)	%	(95% CI)
Sex												
Male	2.8	(2.2–3.6)	4.1	(3.7–4.7)	2.1	(1.8–2.5)	7.7	(7.3–8.2)	4.5	(4.1–4.8)	5.2	(3.5–7.4)
Female	3.1	(2.3–4.1)	3.7	(3.2–4.3)	2.0	(1.7–2.4)	18.2	(17.5–18.9)	12.0	(11.5–12.6)	8.4	(6.4–10.9)
Age group (yrs)												
3–5	—†	—	0.6	(0.2–1.6)	0.5	(0.1–1.6)	NA	NA	NA	NA	NA	NA
6–11	1.7	(1.2–2.4)	2.3	(1.9–2.8)	1.4	(1.0–1.8)	NA	NA	NA	NA	NA	NA
12–17	5.1	(4.1–6.4)	7.1	(6.4–7.8)	3.5	(3.2–4.0)	12.8	(12.4–13.3)	8.1	(7.8–8.5)	6.7	(5.5–8.3)
Race/Ethnicity§												
Hispanic	2.4	(1.7–3.3)	3.9	(2.9–5.2)	1.8	(1.3–2.7)	13.0	(12.0–14.1)	7.9	(7.1–8.8)	5.7	(3.8–8.3)
Black, non-Hispanic	2.5	(1.5–4.1)	3.7	(2.9–4.7)	2.2	(1.5–3.1)	11.1	(10.2–12.2)	6.9	(6.1–7.7)	7.4	(5.5–9.9)
White, non-Hispanic	3.2	(2.5–4.2)	4.0	(3.6–4.5)	2.1	(1.9–2.4)	13.2	(12.7–13.7)	8.6	(8.1–9.0)	7.3	(5.3–10.0)
Multirace, non-Hispanic	8.1¶	(4.3–14.9)¶	5.9	(4.4–7.8)	3.5	(2.4–5.0)	16.2	(13.8–19.0)	10.1	(8.1–12.6)	NA	NA
Other, non-Hispanic	1.5¶	(0.7–3.4)¶	2.6	(1.8–3.7)	1.4	(0.8–2.4)	11.7	(9.7–14.0)	6.7	(5.3–8.4)	NA	NA
Highest education in household**												
Less than high school	5.0	(2.8–8.7)	6.7	(4.9–9.0)	3.4	(2.2–5.2)	NA	NA	NA	NA	6.6	(4.8–9.1)

Table 7. (Continued)

Characteristic	Received a diagnosis of depression during past 12 months (parent report)		Ever received a diagnosis of depression (parent report)		Current depression (parent report)		Lifetime major depressive episode (child report)		Major depressive episode during past 12 months (child report)		Current depression during past 2 weeks (child report, score of ≥10 on PHQ-9)	
	NHIS 2007 Ages: 4–17 years (N = 7,103 persons surveyed)		NSCH 2007 Ages: 3–17 years (N = 78,042 persons surveyed)		NSCH 2007 Ages: 3–17 years (N = 78,042 persons surveyed)		NSDUH 2010–2011 Ages: 12–17 years (N = 45,500 persons surveyed)*		NSDUH 2010–2011 Ages: 12–17 years (N = 45,500 persons surveyed)*		NHANES 2007–2010 Ages: 12–17 years (N = 1,782 persons surveyed)	
	%	(95% CI)	%	(95% CI)	%	(95% CI)	%	(95% CI)	%	(95% CI)	%	(95% CI)
High school graduate	2.7	(1.9–3.7)	5.6	(4.7–6.8)	3.2	(2.6–3.9)	NA	NA	NA	NA	7.0	(4.2–11.4)
More than high school	2.8	(2.2–3.6)	3.1	(2.8–3.5)	1.6	(1.4–1.8)	NA	NA	NA	NA	7.0	(5.0–9.8)
Insurance							NA	NA	NA	NA	NA	NA
Yes	2.9	(2.4–3.6)	3.9	(3.6–4.3)	2.1	(1.9–2.4)	12.7	(12.3–13.1)	8.1	(7.7–8.4)	6.7	(5.3–8.3)
No	3.6	(2.4–5.3)	4.0	(2.7–5.9)	1.8	(1.2–2.7)	14.5	(12.9–16.3)	9.1	(7.8–10.5)	5.3	(8.3–13.9)
Region Northeast	2.3	(1.6–3.5)	3.7	(3.1–4.5)	2.1	(1.6–2.7)	12.1	(11.2–13.1)	7.4	(6.7–8.2)	NA	NA
Midwest	4.0	(2.6–6.2)	4.5	(3.9–5.1)	2.5	(2.1–3.0)	12.5	(11.8–13.2)	8.2	(7.7–8.9)	NA	NA
South	2.8	(2.2–3.7)	3.7	(3.2–4.2)	2.0	(1.6–2.3)	12.9	(12.3–13.6)	8.1	(7.6–8.7)	NA	NA
West	2.6	(1.8–3.6)	4.0	(3.1–5.3)	1.9	(1.3–2.7)	13.6	(12.5–14.7)	8.6	(7.8–9.4)	NA	NA
Poverty-income ratio††												
≤100% FPL	4.4	(3.2–6.0)	6.9	(5.7–8.2)	4.4	(3.5–5.5)	12.4	(11.5–13.3)	7.7	(7.0–8.4)	7.1	(5.3–9.5)
>100% to ≤200% FPL	4.1	(2.6–6.4)	4.6	(3.8–5.6)	2.4	(1.9–3.0)	13.9	(13.0–14.8)	8.9	(8.3–9.7)	8.5	(5.1–13.8)
>200% FPL	2.1	(1.7–2.7)	2.9	(2.5–3.3)	1.3	(1.1–1.6)	12.6	(12.0–13.1)	8.0	(7.5–8.4)	5.9	(4.0–8.7)
Total	3.0	(2.5–3.6)	3.9	(3.6–4.3)	2.1	(1.8–2.4)	12.8	(12.4–13.3)	8.1	(7.8–8.5)	6.7	(5.5–8.3)

Abbreviations: CI = confidence interval; FPL = federal poverty level; NA = not available; NHANES = National Health and Nutrition Examination Survey; NHIS = National Health Interview Survey; NSCH = National Survey of Children's Health; NSDUH = National Survey on Drug Use and Health; PHQ-9 = nine-item Patient Health Questionnaire. * Sample size rounded to the nearest 100 for disclosure reasons.

† Data suppressed because relative standard error is ≥50%.

§ Other, non-Hispanic, includes American Indian/Alaska Native, Hawaiian/other Pacific Islander, and Asian. Persons categorized as multirace selected more than one race. ¶ Relative standard error is >30% and <50%.

** The highest education in the household is based on the highest education of adults in the sample child's family for NHIS and the education of parents or respondents (adults) for NSCH, and the household reference person (usually an adult) for NHANES.

†† FPL is based on family income and family size and composition using federal poverty thresholds that are updated annually by the U.S. Census Bureau using the change in the average annual consumer price index for all urban consumers. (Additional information available at http://www.census.gov/hhes/www/poverty/index.html.)

Table 8. Prevalence of children aged 3–17 years who had phobias or fears in the past 12 months, ever received a diagnosis of anxiety, or had current anxiety, by sociodemographic characteristics — National Health Interview Survey and National Survey of Children's Health, United States, 2007

	Phobias or fears during past 12 months (parent report)		Ever received a diagnosis of anxiety (parent report)		Current anxiety (in addition to previous diagnosis of anxiety) (parent report)	
	NHIS 2007		NSCH 2007		NSCH 2007	
	Ages: 4–17 years (N = 7,103 persons surveyed)		Ages: 3–17 years (N = 78,042 persons surveyed)		Ages: 3–17 years (N = 78,042 persons surveyed)	
Characteristic	%	(95% CI)	%	(95% CI)	%	(95% CI)
Sex						
Male	2.4	(1.9–3.1)	5.0	(4.6–5.6)	3.4	(3.0–3.8)
Female	2.9	(2.3–3.6)	4.4	(3.8–5.0)	2.6	(2.3–3.0)
Age group (yrs) 2–5	2.6	(1.6–4.1)	1.5	(1.0–2.4)	1.0	(0.7–1.4)
6–11	2.9	(2.3–3.7)	4.3	(3.8–5.0)	2.9	(2.5–3.4)
12–17	2.4	(1.9–3.1)	6.6	(6.0–7.3)	4.1	(3.6–4.6)
Race/Ethnicity*						
Hispanic	2.5	(1.8–3.4)	4.6	(3.5–6.0)	2.6	(1.8–3.6)
Black, non-Hispanic	3.0	(1.9–4.6)	3.3	(2.6–4.2)	2.2	(1.6–3.0)
White, non-Hispanic	2.6	(2.1–3.3)	5.2	(4.8–5.6)	3.4	(3.1–3.7)

Table 8. (Continued)

Characteristic	Phobias or fears during past 12 months (parent report)		Ever received a diagnosis of anxiety (parent report)		Current anxiety (in addition to previous diagnosis of anxiety) (parent report)	
	NHIS 2007		NSCH 2007		NSCH 2007	
	Ages: 4–17 years (N = 7,103 persons surveyed)		Ages: 3–17 years (N = 78,042 persons surveyed)		Ages: 3–17 years (N = 78,042 persons surveyed)	
	%	(95% CI)	%	(95% CI)	%	(95% CI)
Multirace, non-Hispanic	5.5†	(2.6–11.2)†	6.4	(4.8–8.4)	4.7	(3.3–6.6)
Other, non-Hispanic	1.0†	(0.4–2.6)†	2.8	(2.0–3.9)	2.0	(1.3–3.0)
Highest education in household§						
Less than high school	3.6	(2.4–5.6)	6.1	(4.3–8.4)	3.4	(2.4–4.9)
High school graduate	2.6	(1.8–3.6)	4.8	(4.0–5.8)	3.4	(2.8–4.3)
More than high school	2.5	(2.1–3.1)	4.6	(4.2–5.0)	2.9	(2.6–3.2)
Health insurance						
Yes	2.5	(2.1–3.0)	4.9	(4.5–5.3)	3.1	(2.9–3.5)
No	3.6	(2.2–5.8)	3.3	(2.2–4.9)	1.7	(1.2–2.3)
Region Northeast	2.3	(1.5–3.4)	5.1	(4.5–5.8)	3.2	(2.7–3.8)
Midwest	2.1	(1.5–3.1)	5.1	(4.5–5.7)	3.5	(3.0–4.1)
South	2.8	(2.1–3.8)	4.4	(4.0–5.0)	2.9	(2.5–3.3)
West	3.2	(2.3–4.3)	4.6	(3.5–5.9)	2.6	(1.9–3.5)
Poverty-income ratio¶						
≤100% FPL	4.0	(2.8–5.8)	6.3	(5.3–7.4)	4.2	(3.5–5.0)
>100% to ≤200% FPL	2.4	(1.7–3.5)	5.2	(4.2–6.3)	3.5	(2.8–4.5)

Characteristic	Phobias or fears during past 12 months (parent report)		Ever received a diagnosis of anxiety (parent report)		Current anxiety (in addition to previous diagnosis of anxiety) (parent report)	
	NHIS 2007		NSCH 2007		NSCH 2007	
	Ages: 4–17 years (N = 7,103 persons surveyed)		Ages: 3–17 years (N = 78,042 persons surveyed)		Ages: 3–17 years (N = 78,042 persons surveyed)	
	%	(95% CI)	%	(95% CI)	%	(95% CI)
>200% FPL	2.3	(1.9–2.9)	4.1	(3.7–4.6)	2.5	(2.2–2.8)
Total	2.6	(2.2–3.1)	4.7	(4.4–5.1)	3.0	(2.7–3.3)

Abbreviations: CI = confidence interval; FPL = federal poverty level; NSCH, National Survey of Children's Health; NHIS = National Health Interview Survey. * Other, non-Hispanic, includes American Indian/Alaska Native, Hawaiian/other Pacific Islander, and Asian. Persons categorized as multirace selected more than one race.

† Relative standard error is >30% and <50%.

§ The highest education in the household is based on the highest education of adults in the sample child's family for NHIS and the education of parents or respondents (adults) for NSCH.

¶ FPL is based on family income and family size and composition using federal poverty thresholds that are updated annually by the U.S. Census Bureau using the change in the average annual consumer price index for all urban consumers. (Additional information available at http://www.census.gov/ hhes/www/poverty/index.html.)

Table 9. Prevalence of adolescents aged 12–17 years who reported having had an alcohol use disorder or illicit drug use disorder in the past year, dependence on cigarettes in the past month, alcohol or illicit drug use in the past year, or cigarettes use in the past month, by sociodemographic characteristics — National Survey on Drug Use and Health,* United States, 2010–2011

Characteristic	Past year alcohol use disorder†		Past year illicit drug use disorder§		Past month cigarette dependence¶		Past year alcohol use		Past year illicit drug use		Past month cigarette use	
	%	(95% CI)	%	(95% CI)	%	(95% CI)	%	(95% CI)	%	(95% CI)	%	(95% CI)

Table 9. (Continued)

Characteristic	Past year alcohol use disorder†		Past year illicit drug use disorder§		Past month cigarette dependence¶		Past year alcohol use		Past year illicit drug use		Past month cigarette use	
	%	(95% CI)	%	(95% CI)	%	(95% CI)	%	(95% CI)	%	(95% CI)	%	(95% CI)
Sex												
Male	3.7	(3.4–4.0)	4.8	(4.4–5.2)	3.0	(2.8–3.4)	27.4	(26.6–28.2)	19.3	(18.5–20.0)	8.4	(7.9–8.9)
Female	4.7	(4.3–5.1)	4.6	(4.2–5.0)	2.5	(2.3–2.8)	29.1	(28.3–29.9)	19.2	(18.5–19.9)	7.7	(7.3–8.2)
Race/Ethnicity**												
Hispanic	4.5	(4.0–5.2)	5.7	(5.0–6.4)	1.8	(1.4–2.3)	28.5	(27.1–29.8)	20.9	(19.8–22.1)	6.9	(6.2–7.8)
Black, non-Hispanic	2.4	(1.9–3.0)	4.1	(3.5–4.8)	1.6	(1.2–2.0)	23.7	(22.3–25.2)	19.6	(18.4–20.9)	4.7	(4.0–5.4)
White, non-Hispanic	4.6	(4.2–4.9)	4.6	(4.2–4.9)	3.6	(3.3–3.9)	30.0	(29.3–30.7)	18.9	(18.3–19.5)	9.6	(9.1–10.1)
Multirace, non-Hispanic	5.6	(4.2–7.5)	6.4	(4.8–8.5)	4.1	(2.7–6.0)	32.7	(29.2–36.4)	26.7	(23.4–30.3)	10.0	(7.9–12.6)
Other, non-Hispanic	2.7	(2.0–3.7)	2.8	(2.0–3.9)	1.2	(0.8–2.0)	18.6	(16.4–21.1)	11.6	(9.9–13.7)	4.5	(3.4–5.9)
Insurance												
Yes	4.0	(3.8–4.3)	4.7	(4.4–4.9)	2.7	(2.5–3.0)	28.0	(27.4–28.6)	19.0	(18.5–19.5)	7.8	(7.5–8.2)
No	5.9	(4.8–7.2)	5.1	(4.2–6.3)	3.7	(2.9–4.6)	31.1	(28.9–33.4)	22.2	(20.3–24.3)	11.0	(9.5–12.8)
Region Northeast	4.4	(3.9–5.0)	4.7	(4.1–5.3)	2.7	(2.3–3.3)	32.3	(31.0–33.6)	19.9	(18.8–21.0)	8.2	(7.5–9.0)
Midwest	3.8	(3.4–4.2)	4.3	(3.9–4.7)	3.5	(3.0–4.0)	27.8	(26.8–28.8)	18.1	(17.3–18.9)	8.7	(8.0–9.4)
South	3.7	(3.3–4.1)	4.2	(3.7–4.6)	2.8	(2.5–3.2)	26.8	(25.8–27.8)	17.8	(16.9–18.7)	8.0	(7.4–8.6)
West	5.2	(4.5–5.8)	5.9	(5.3–6.6)	2.2	(1.8–2.6)	27.9	(26.5–29.4)	22.0	(20.7–23.3)	7.5	(6.8–8.3)
Poverty-income ratio††												
≤100% FPL	4.4	(3.8–5.0)	5.7	(5.0–6.4)	3.9	(3.4–4.4)	26.0	(24.7–27.4)	20.7	(19.6–22.0)	9.2	(8.5–10.0)
>100% to ≤200% FPL	4.0	(3.5–4.6)	4.9	(4.4–5.5)	3.4	(2.9–3.9)	27.2	(26.0–28.3)	19.8	(18.8–20.9)	8.9	(8.2–9.8)
>200% FPL	4.2	(3.8–4.5)	4.2	(3.9–4.6)	2.1	(1.9–2.4)	29.5	(28.7–30.3)	18.4	(17.7–19.1)	7.3	(6.8–7.7)
Total	4.2	(3.9–4.4)	4.7	(4.4–5.0)	2.8	(2.6–3.0)	28.2	(27.7–28.8)	19.2	(18.7–19.7)	8.1	(7.7–8.4)

Abbreviations: CI = confidence interval; DSM-IV = Diagnostic and Statistical Manual of Mental Disorders, Fourth Edition; FPL = federal poverty level; NSDUH = National Survey on Drug Use and Health.

* N ≈ 45,500 surveys. Sample size rounded to the nearest 100 for disclosure reasons.

† Alcohol use disorder is defined as alcohol dependence or abuse, based on definitions found in DSM-IV. (Source: American Psychiatric Association. Diagnostic and statistical manual of mental disorders. 4th ed, text revision. Washington, DC: American Psychiatric Association; 2000.)

§ Illicit drug use disorder is defined as illicit drug dependence or abuse, based on definitions found in DSM-IV. Illicit drugs include marijuana/hashish, cocaine (including crack), heroin, hallucinogens, inhalants, or prescription-type psychotherapeutics used nonmedically, including data from original methamphetamine questions but not including new methamphetamine items added in 2005 and 2006.

¶ Nicotine (cigarette) dependence is based on criteria from the Nicotine Dependence Syndrome Scale or the Fagerstrom Test of Nicotine Dependence. (Source: Substance Abuse and Mental Health Services Administration. Results from the 2009 National Survey on Drug Use and Health. Vol II. Technical appendices and selected prevalence tables. Rockville, MD: US Department of Health and Human Services; 2010.)

** Other, non-Hispanic, includes American Indian/Alaska Native, Hawaiian/other Pacific Islander, and Asian. Persons categorized as multirace selected more than one race. †† FPL is based on family income and family size and composition using federal poverty thresholds that are updated annually by the U.S. Census Bureau using the change in the average annual consumer price index for all urban consumers. (Additional information available at http://www.census.gov/hhes/www/poverty/index.html.)

Table 10. Prevalence of adolescents aged 12–17 years who reported ≥14 mentally unhealthy days in the past month, by sociodemographic characteristics and year — National Health and Nutrition Examination Survey,* United States, 2005–2010

Characteristic	%	(95% CI)
Sex		
Male	6.7	(4.7–8.7)
Female	10.0	(8.0–12.1)
Race/Ethnicity† Mexican-American	4.9	(3.3–6.6)
Black, non-Hispanic	6.6	(4.9–8.3)

Table 10. (Continued)

Characteristic	%	(95% CI)
White, non-Hispanic	9.6	(7.5–11.8)
Education of household reference person§		
Less than high school	5.9	(4.3–7.4)
High school graduate	9.6	(5.7–13.4)
More than high school	8.7	(6.9–10.5)
Health insurance		
Yes	8.2	(6.7–9.7)
No	9.8	(4.7–14.8)
Poverty-income ratio¶		
≤100% FPL	8.1	(5.3–10.9)
>100% to ≤200% FPL	10.5	(7.5–13.5)
>200% FPL	7.6	(5.8–9.3)
Total	8.3	(6.9–9.8)

Abbreviations: CI = confidence interval; FPL = federal poverty level; NHANES = National Health and Nutrition Examination Survey.

* N = 3,312 surveys.

† Persons of other race not presented because of the small sample size.

§ The highest education in the household is based on the household reference person (usually an adult) for NHANES.

¶ FPL is based on family income and family size and composition using federal poverty thresholds that are updated annually by the U.S. Census Bureau using the change in the average annual consumer price index for all urban consumers. (Additional information available at http://www.census.gov/hhes/www/poverty/ index.html.)

Table 11. Number and rate of suicide deaths among persons aged 10–19 years, by sociodemographic characteristics, mechanism of death, and known circumstances — National Vital Statistics System, United States, 2010, and National Violent Death Reporting System, 16 states,* 2005–2009

	NVSS 2010		NVDRS 2005–2009										
	Suicide deaths		Suicide deaths		Suicide deaths with known circumstances†								
					Total	Previous suicide attempt		Disclosed intent to commit suicide		Current mental disorder		Current mental disorder treatment	
Characteristic	No.	Rate§	No.	Rate§	Total	No.	%	No.	%	No.	%	No.	%
Sex													
Male	1,503	6.9	1,890	6.54	1570	263	16.8	457	29.1	508	32.4	369	23.5
Female	423	2.0	500	1.83	451	163	36.1	140	31	210	46.6	165	36.6
Age group (yrs)¶													
10–14	267	1.3	302	1.13	255	50	19.6	76	29.8	90	35.3	65	25.5
15–19	1,659	7.5	2,088	7.39	1766	376	21.3	521	29.5	628	35.6	469	26.6
Race/Ethnicity**													
Hispanic	295	3.3	234	3.81	201	48	23.9	68	33.8	54	26.9	41	20.4
Black, non-Hispanic	189	2.8	280	2.64	206	29	14.1	47	22.8	64	31.1	40	19.4
White, non-Hispanic	1,299	5.3	1,658	4.51	1427	310	21.7	427	29.2	543	38.1	412	28.9
Other, non-Hispanic	135	5.3	188	8.46	158	35	22.2	50	31.7	46	29.1	36	22.8
Mechanism													
Poisoning	121	0.3	145	0.26	—††	—††	—††	—††	—††	—††	—††	—††	—††
Hanging/Suffocation	920	2.2	1,082	1.93	—††	—††	—††	—††	—††	—††	—††	—††	—††

Table 11. (Continued)

	NVSS 2010		NVDRS 2005–2009										
	Suicide deaths		Suicide deaths		Suicide deaths with known circumstances†								
					Total	Previous suicide attempt		Disclosed intent to commit suicide		Current mental disorder		Current mental disorder treatment	
Characteristic	No.	Rate§	No.	Rate§	Total	No.	%	No.	%	No.	%	No.	%
Motor vehicle			58	0.10	—††	—††	—††	—††	—††	—††	—††	—††	—††
Firearm	748	1.8	1,024	1.81	—††	—††	—††	—††	—††	—††	—††	—††	—††
Other/Unknown	137	0.3	81	—§§	—††	—††	—††	—††	—††	—††	—††	—††	—††
Total	1,926	4.5	2,390	4.24	2021	426	21.1	597	29.5	718	35.5	534	26.4

Abbreviations: NVDRS = National Violent Death Reporting System; NVSS = National Vital Statistics System.

* Alaska, Colorado, Georgia, Kentucky, Maryland, Massachusetts, New Jersey, New Mexico, North Carolina, Oklahoma, Oregon, Rhode Island, South Carolina, Utah, Virginia, and Wisconsin.

† Decedents can have one or more circumstances; therefore, subcategories might not sum to all known circumstances.

§ Rate per 100,000 children; all rates are age adjusted using the 2000 U.S. standard population (all races, both sexes).

¶ Suicide among children aged ≤9 years are suppressed in NVDRS reporting on the basis of a child's inability to form and understand suicidal intent and consequences.

** Other, non-Hispanic, includes American Indian/Alaska Native, Hawaiian/other Pacific Islander, and Asian.

†† Data available from restricted access dataset only. Data presented in this table were obtained using WISQARS.

§§ Rates based on these numbers from cell sizes <20 have been suppressed because they might be unstable.

ACKNOWLEDGMENTS

This report is based, in part, on contributions by William Beardslee, MD, Harvard Medical School, Boston, Massachusetts; Melissa L. Brodowski, PhD, Children's Bureau, Administration for Children and Families, Washington, DC; Ileana Arias, PhD, Office of the Director, Stephen B. Thacker (deceased), Office of Science, Epidemiology, and Laboratory Services, Coleen A. Boyle, PhD, Marshalyn Yeargin-Allsopp, MD, Jacquelyn Bertrand, PhD, Joseph Holbrook, PhD, Emily Deubler, National Center on Birth Defects and Developmental Disabilities, Deborah Gould, PhD, Public Health Surveillance Program Office, Wanjun Cui, PhD, National Center for Chronic Disease Prevention and Health Promotion, CDC, Atlanta, Georgia; and Margaret Warner, PhD, National Center for Health Statistics, CDC, Hyattsville, Maryland.

REFERENCES

[1] Lippman LH, Moore KA, McIntosh H. Positive indicators of child well-being: a conceptual framework, measures, and methodological issues. *Appl. Res. Qual. Life* 2011;6:425–49.

[2] Hoagwood K, Jensen PS, Petti T, Burns BJ. Outcomes of mental health care for children and adolescents: I. A comprehensive conceptual model. *J. Am. Acad. Child Adolesc. Psychiatry* 1996;35:1055–63.

[3] World Health Organization. Mental health policy and service guidance package: child and adolescent mental health policies and plans. Geneva, Switzerland: World Health Organization; 2005.

[4] US Department of Health and Human Services Health Resources and Services Administration & Maternal and Child Health Bureau. Mental health: A report of the Surgeon General. Rockville, MD: US Department of Health and Human Services, Substance Abuse and Mental Health Services Administration, Center for Mental Health Services, and National Institutes of Health, National Institute of Mental Health; 1999.

[5] American Psychiatric Association. Diagnostic and statistical manual of mental disorders. 4th ed, text revision. Washington, DC: American Psychiatric Association; 2000.

[6] National Research Council and Institute of Medicine. Preventing mental, emotional, and behavioral disorders among young people: progress and possibilities. Washington, DC: The National Academic Press; 2009.
[7] World Health Organization. International statistical classification of diseases and related health problems, ICD–10. Geneva, Switzerland: World Health Organization; 1992.
[8] Angold A, Erkanli A, Farmer EM, et al. Psychiatric disorder, impairment, and service use in rural African American and white youth. *Arch. Gen. Psychiatry* 2002;59:893–901.
[9] Merikangas KR, He JP, Brody D, Fisher PW, Bourdon K, Koretz DS. Prevalence and treatment of mental disorders among U.S. children in the 2001–2004 NHANES. *Pediatrics* 2010;125:75–81.
[10] World Health Organization. Mental health: a state of well-being. Geneva, Switzerland: World Health Organization; 2011. Available at http://www. who.int/features/factfiles/mental_health/en/index.html.
[11] CDC. Web-Based Injury Statistics Query and Reporting System (WISQARS). Atlanta, GA; 2011. Available at http://www.cdc.gov/ injury/wisqars/index.html.
[12] Eisenberg D, Neighbors K. Economic and policy issues in preventing mental disorders and substance abuse among young people: presentation for the IOM Committee on the Prevention of Mental Disorders and Substance Abuse, October 31st, 2007: Department of Health Management and Policy School of Public Health, University of Michigan; 2007.
[13] Kogan MD, Strickland BB, Blumberg SJ, Singh GK, Perrin JM, van Dyck PC. A national profile of the health care experiences and family impact of autism spectrum disorder among children in the United States, 2005–2006. *Pediatrics* 2008;122:e1149–58.
[14] Soni A. The five most costly children's conditions, 2006: estimates for the U.S. civilian noninstitutionalized children, ages 0–17. Rockville, MD: Agency for Healthcare Research and Quality; 2009. April Contract No.: Statistical Brief #242.
[15] Health Care Cost Institute. Children's health care spending report: 2007–2010. Washington, DC: Health Care Cost Institute; 2012.
[16] Pfuntner A, Wier LM, Stocks C. Most frequent conditions in U.S. hospitals, 2010 Rockville, MD: Agency for Healthcare Research and Quality; 2013. January Contract No.: HCUP Statistical Brief #148.

[17] Kessler RC, Foster CL, Saunders WB, Stang PE. Social-consequences of psychiatric-disorders. 1. educational-attainment. *Am. J. Psychiatry* 1995;152:1026–32.

[18] Lewinsohn PM, Rohde P, Seeley JR. Major depressive disorder in older adolescents: prevalence, risk factors, and clinical implications. *Clin. Psychol. Rev.* 1998;18:765–94.

[19] Schieve LA, Boulet SL, Kogan MD, et al. Parenting aggravation and autism spectrum disorders: 2007 National Survey of Children's Health. *Disabil. Health J.* 2011;4:143–52.

[20] Copeland WE, Miller-Johnson S, Keeler G, Angold A, Costello EJ. Childhood psychiatric disorders and young adult crime: a prospective, population-based study. *Am. J. Psychiatry* 2007;164:1668–75.

[21] Lehrer JA, Shrier LA, Gortmaker S, Buka S. Depressive symptoms as a longitudinal predictor of sexual risk behaviors among U.S. middle and high school students. *Pediatrics* 2006;118:189–200.

[22] Substance Abuse and Mental Health Services Administration. The NSDUH report: major depressive episode among youths aged 12 to 17 in the United States: 2004 to 2006. Rockville, MD: Office of Applied Studies; 2008.

[23] Costello EJ, Mustillo S, Erkanli A, Keeler G, Angold A. Prevalence and development of psychiatric disorders in childhood and adolescence. *Arch. Gen. Psychiatry* 2003;60:837–44.

[24] Kessler RC, Avenevoli S, McLaughlin KA, et al. Lifetime co-morbidity of DSM-IV disorders in the US National Comorbidity Survey Replication Adolescent Supplement (NCS-A). *Psychol. Med.* 2012;42:1997–2010.

[25] Merikangas KR, He JP, Burstein M, et al. Lifetime prevalence of mental disorders in U.S. adolescents: results from the National Comorbidity Survey Replication—Adolescent Supplement (NCS-A). *J. Am. Acad. Child Adolesc. Psychiatry* 2010;49:980–9.

[26] US Department ofHealth and Human Services, Health Resources and Services Administration, Maternal and Child Health Bureau. The mental and emotional well-being of children: a portrait of states and the nation 2007. Rockville, MD: US Department of Health and Human Services; 2010.

[27] Delmas MC, Guignon N, Chee CC, Fuhrman C, Herbet JB, Gonzalez L. Asthma and major depressive episode in adolescents in France. *J. Asthma* 2011;48:640–6.

[28] Reilly C, Agnew R, Neville BG. Depression and anxiety in childhood epilepsy: a review. *Seizure* 2011;20:589–97.

[29] Roy-Byrne PP, Davidson KW, Kessler RC, et al. Anxiety disorders and comorbid medical illness. *Gen. Hosp. Psychiatry* 2008;30:208–25.

[30] Shomaker LB, Tanofsky-Kraff M, Stern EA, et al. Longitudinal study of depressive symptoms and progression of insulin resistance in youth at risk for adult obesity. *Diabetes Care* 2011;34:2458–63.

[31] CDC. Mental illness surveillance among adults in the United States. *MMWR* 2011;60(Suppl).

[32] Smit F, Cuijpers P, Oostenbrink J, Batelaan N, de Graaf R, Beekman A. Costs of nine common mental disorders: implications for curative and preventive psychiatry. *J. Ment. Health Policy Econ.* 2006;9:193–200.

[33] CDC. Updated guidelines for evaluating public health surveillance systems. *MMWR* 2001;50(No. RR-13):1–35.

[34] CDC. CDC's vision for public health surveillance in the 21st century. MMWR 2012;61(Suppl).

[35] Thacker SB. Historical development. In: Teutsch SM, Churchill RE, eds. Principles and practice of public health surveillance. 2nd ed. New York, NY: Oxford University Press; 2000.

[36] Substance Abuse and Mental Health Services Administration. Mental health, United States, 2010. Rockville, MD: Substance Abuse and Mental Health Services Administration; 2012. http://www.samhsa.gov/data/2k12/MHUS2010/index.aspx.

[37] Miles J, Espiritu RC, Horen N, Sebian J, Waetzing E. A public health approach to children's mental health: a conceptual framework. Washington, DC: Georgetown University Center for Child and Human Development, National Technical Assistance Center for Children's Mental Health; 2010.

[38] Hedden S, Gfroerer J, Barker P, et al. CBHSQ data review: comparison of NSDUH mental health data and methods with other data sources: Center for Behavioral Health Statistics and Quality, Substance Abuse and Mental Health Services Administration; 2012.

[39] Kessler RC, Avenevoli S, Costello EJ, et al. Design and field procedures in the U.S. National Comorbidity Survey Replication Adolescent Supplement (NCS-A). *Int. J. Methods Psychiatr. Res*. 2009;18:69–83.

[40] Merikangas K, Avenevoli S, Costello J, Koretz D, Kessler RC. National comorbidity survey replication adolescent supplement (NCS-A): I. Background and measures. *J. Am. Acad. Child Adolesc. Psychiatry* 2009;48:367–9.

[41] Yeargin-Allsopp M, Rice C, Karapurkar T, Doernberg N, Boyle C, Murphy C. Prevalence of autism in a U.S. metropolitan area. *JAMA* 2003;289:49–55.

[42] Rice CE, Baio J, Van Naarden Braun K, et al. A public health collaboration for the surveillance of autism spectrum disorders. *Paediatr. Perinat. Epidemiol.* 2007;21:179–90.

[43] National Center for Health Statistics. Bridged-race population estimates data files and documentation 2010. Estimates of the United States resident population from the vintage 2009 postcensal series by year, county, age, sex, race, and Hispanic origin. Hyattsville, MD: CDC, US Department of Health and Human Services. Available at http://www.cdc.gov/nchs/ nvss/bridged_race/data_documentation.htm#vintage2009.

[44] CDC. *National Health and Nutrition Examination Survey* (NHANES). Atlanta, GA: CDC. Available at http://www.cdc.gov/nchs/nhanes.htm.

[45] Shaffer D, Fisher P, Lucas CP, Dulcan MK, Schwab-Stone ME. NIMH Diagnostic Interview Schedule for Children Version IV (NIMH DISC-IV): description, differences from previous versions, and reliability of some common diagnoses. *J. Am. Acad. Child Adolesc. Psychiatry* 2000;39:28–38.

[46] Richardson LP, McCauley E, Grossman DC, et al. Evaluation of the Patient Health Questionnaire–9 Item for detecting major depression among adolescents. *Pediatrics* 2010;126:1117–23.

[47] Spitzer R, Kroenke K, William J. Validation and utility of a self-report version of PRIME-MD: the PHQ primary care study. Primary care evaluation of mental disorders. Patient health questionnaire. *JAMA* 1999;282:1737–44.

[48] Dube S, Thompson WW, Homa D, Zack M. Association between smoking behaviors and health-related quality of life among adolescents aged 12–17 years. *Nicotine & Tobacco Control.* 2013;15:492–500.

[49] Zullig KJ, Valois RF, Huebner ES, Drane JW. Evaluating the performance of the Centers for Disease Control and Prevention core Health-Related Quality of Life scale with adolescents. *Public Health Rep.* 2004;119:577–84.

[50] Zullig KJ, Valois RF, Huebner ES, Drane JW. Adolescent health-related quality of life and perceived satisfaction with life. *Qual. Life Res.* 2005;14:1573–84.

[51] CDC; National Center for Health Statistics. National Health Interview Survey. Atlanta, GA: CDC; 2012. Available at http://www.cdc.gov/nchs/ nhis.htm.

[52] Achenbach T. Manual for the child behavior checklist/2-3 and 1992 profile. Burlington, VT: University of Vermont Department of Psychiatry; 1992.

[53] Goodman A, Goodman R. Strengths and difficulties questionnaire as a dimensional measure of child mental health. *J. Am. Acad. Child Adolesc. Psychiatry* 2009;48:400–3.

[54] Goodman R. The strengths and difficulties questionnaire: a research note. *J. Child Psychol. Psychiatry* 1997;38:581–6.

[55] Blumberg SJ, Foster EB, Frasier AM, et al. Design and operation of the National Survey of Children's Health, 2007. Hyattsville, MD: *National Center for Health Statistics*; 2009.

[56] American Academy of Family Physicians, American Academy of Pediatrics, American College of Physicians, American Osteopathic Association. Joint principles of the patient centered medical home; 2007. Available at http:// www.pcpcc.net/content/joint-principles-patient-centered-medical-home.

[57] Substance Abuse and Mental Health Services Administration. Results from the 2010 National Survey on Drug Use and Health: mental health findings. NSDUH Series H-42, HHS Publication No. (SMA) 11-4667. Rockville, MD: Substance *Abuse and Mental Health Services Administration*; 2012.

[58] Dahlberg LL, Krug EG. Violence—a global public health problem. Geneva, Switzerland: World Health Organization; 2002.

[59] Paulozzi LJ, Mercy J, Frazier L, Annest JL. CDC's National Violent Death Reporting System: background and methodology. *Inj. Prev.* 2004;10:47–52.

[60] Kochanek KD, Xu JQ, Murphy SL, Miniño AM, Kun HC. Deaths: final data for 2009. Natl Vital Stat Rep 2011;60.

[61] CDC. CDC WONDER. Atlanta, GA: CDC; 2013. Available at http://wonder.cdc.gov.

[62] CDC. School associated violent death study. Atlanta, GA: CDC; 2010. Available at http://www.cdc.gov/violenceprevention/youthviolence/schoolviolence/SAVD.html.

[63] CDC. Methodology of the Youth Risk Behavior Surveillance System—2013. *MMWR* 2013;66(No. RR-1).

[64] CDC. Youth risk behavior surveillance—United States, 2011. MMWR 2012;61(No. SS-4).

[65] Larson K, Russ SA, Kahn RS, Halfon N. Patterns of comorbidity, functioning, and service use for U.S. children with ADHD, 2007. *Pediatrics* 2011;127:462–70.

[66] Loe I, Feldman H. Academic and educational outcomes of children with ADHD. *J. Pediatr. Psychol.* 2007;32:643–54.

[67] Nijmeijer JS, Minderaa RB, Buitelaar JK, Mulligan A, Hartman CA, Hoekstra PJ. Attention-deficit/hyperactivity disorder and social dysfunctioning. *Clin. Psychol. Rev.* 2008;28:692–708.

[68] Charach A, Yeung E, Climans T, Lillie E. Childhood attention-deficit/hyperactivity disorder and future substance use disorders: comparative meta-analyses. *J. Am. Acad. Child Adolesc. Psychiatry* 2011;50:9–21.

[69] DeWolfe N, Byrne JM, Bawden HN. ADHD in preschool children: parent-rated psychosocial correlates. *Dev. Med. Child Neurol.* 2000; 42:825–30.

[70] Lee SS, Humphreys KL, Flory K, Liu R, Glass K. Prospective association of childhood attention-deficit/hyperactivity disorder (ADHD) and substance use and abuse/dependence: a meta-analytic review. *Clin. Psychol. Rev.* 2011;31:328–41.

[71] Merrill R, Lyon J, Baker R, Gren L. Attention deficit hyperactivity disorder and increased risk of injury. *Adv. Med. Sci.* 2009;54:20–6.

[72] Molina BS, Pelham WE, Gnagy EM, Thompson AL, Marshal MP. Attention-deficit/hyperactivity disorder risk for heavy drinking and alcohol use disorder is age specific. *Alcohol. Clin. Exp. Res.* 2007; 31:643–54.

[73] Pastor PN, Reuben CA. Identified attention-deficit/hyperactivity disorder and medically attended, nonfatal injuries: U.S. school-age children, 1997–2002. *Ambul. Pediatr.* 2006;6:38–44.

[74] Schwebel DC, Roth DL, Elliott MN, et al. Association of externalizing behavior disorder symptoms and injury among fifth graders. *Acad. Pediatr.* 2011;11:427–31.

[75] Wilens TE, Vitulano M, Upadhyaya H, et al. Cigarette smoking associated with attention deficit hyperactivity disorder. *J. Pediatr.* 2008;153:414–9.

[76] Froehlich TE, Lanphear BP, Epstein JN, Barbaresi WJ, Katusic SK, Kahn RS. Prevalence, recognition, and treatment of attention-deficit/hyperactivity disorder in a national sample of U.S. children. *Arch. Pediatr. Adolesc. Med.* 2007;161:857–64.

[77] Biederman J, Petty CR, Dolan C, et al. The long-term longitudinal course of oppositional defiant disorder and conduct disorder in ADHD

boys: findings from a controlled 10-year prospective longitudinal follow-up study. *Psychol. Med.* 2008;38:1027–36.

[78] Gurney JG, McPheeters ML, Davis MM. Parental report of health conditions and health care use among children with and without autism—National Survey of Children's Health. *Arch. Pediatr. Adolesc. Med.* 2006;160:825–30.

[79] Levy SE, Giarelli E, Lee LC, et al. Autism spectrum disorder and co-occurring developmental, psychiatric, and medical conditions among children in multiple populations of the United States. *J. Dev. Behav. Pediatr.* 2010;31:267–75.

[80] Schieve LA, Gonzalez V, Boulet SL, et al. Concurrent medical conditions and health care use and needs among children with learning and behavioral developmental disabilities, National Health Interview Survey, 2006–2010. *Res. Dev. Disabil.* 2012;33:467–76.

[81] Bitsko RH, Visser SN, Schieve LA, Ross DS, Thurman DJ, Perou R. Unmet health care needs among CSHCN with neurologic conditions. *Pediatrics* 2009;124(Suppl 4):S343–51.

[82] Boyle CA, Boulet S, Schieve LA, et al. Trends in the prevalence of developmental disabilities in U.S. children, 1997–2008. *Pediatrics* 2011;127:1034–42.

[83] Fombonne E. Past and future perspectives on autism epidemiology. In: Moldin SO, Rubenstein JLR, ed. Understanding autism: from basic neuroscience to treatment. Boca Raton, FL: Taylor and Francis Group; 2006.

[84] Schieve LA, Rice C, Devine O, et al. Have secular changes in perinatal risk factors contributed to the recent autism prevalence increase? Development and application of a mathematical assessment model. *Ann. Epidemiol.* 2011;21:930–45.

[85] CDC. Parental report of diagnosed autism in children aged 4–17 years—United States, 2003–2004. *MMWR* 2006;55:481–6.

[86] American Psychiatric Association. Diagnostic and statistical manual of mental disorders. 4th ed. Washington, DC: American Psychiatric Association; 1994.

[87] 87 Angold A, Costello EJ, Erkanli A. Comorbidity. *J. Child Psychol. Psychiatry* 1999;40:57–87.

[88] Kessler RC, Berglund P, Demler O, Jin R, Walters EE. Lifetime prevalence and age-of-onset distributions' of DSM-IV disorders in the national comorbidity survey replication. *Arch. Gen. Psychiatry* 2005;62:593–602.

[89] Pinquart M, Shen Y. Depressive symptoms in children and adolescents with chronic physical illness: an updated meta-analysis. *J. Pediatr. Psychol.* 2011;36:375–84.

[90] Crum RM, Green KM, Storr CL, et al. Depressed mood in childhood and subsequent alcohol use through adolescence and young adulthood. *Arch. Gen. Psychiatry* 2008;65:702–12.

[91] Audrain-McGovern J, Rodriguez D, Kassel JD. Adolescent smoking and depression: evidence for self-medication and peer smoking mediation. *Addiction* 2009;104:1743–56.

[92] Armstrong TD, Costello EJ. Community studies on adolescent substance use, abuse, or dependence and psychiatric comorbidity. *J. Consult. Clin. Psychol.* 2002;70:1224–39.

[93] Lewinsohn PM, Klein DN, Seeley JR. Bipolar disorder during adolescence and young adulthood in a community sample. *Bipolar Disord.* 2000;2:281–93.

[94] Weissman MM, Wolk S, Wickramaratne P, et al. Children with prepubertal-onset major depressive disorder and anxiety grown up. *Arch. Gen. Psychiatry* 1999;56:794–801.

[95] Kessler RC, Walters EE, Forthofer MS. The social consequences of psychiatric disorders, III: Probability of marital stability. *Am. J. Psychiatry* 1998;155:1092–6.

[96] Kennet J, Gfroerer J. Evaluating and improving methods used in the National Survey on Drug Use and Health. Rockville, MD: Substance Abuse and Mental Health Services Administration, Office of Applied Studies 2005 Contract No.: DHHS Publication No. *SMA* 05-4044, Methodology Series M-5.

[97] Substance Abuse and Mental Health Services Administration. Results from the 2011 National Survey on Drug Use and Health: Mental Health Findings and Detailed Tables Rockville, MD: Substance Abuse and Mental Health Services Administration; 2012. Available at http://www.samhsa. gov/data/NSDUH/2k11MH_FindingsandDetTables/Index.aspx.

[98] CDC. Youth risk behavior surveillance—United States, 2009. MMWR 2010;59(No. SS-5).

[99] Wade TJ, Cairney J, Pevalin DJ. Emergence of gender differences in depression during adolescence: national panel results from three countries. *J. Am. Acad. Child Adolesc. Psychiatry* 2002;41:190–8.

[100] Han B, Gfroerer JC, Colliver JD. Associations between duration of illicit drug use and health conditions: results from the 2005–2007 National Surveys on Drug Use and Health. *Ann. Epidemiol.* 2010; 20:289–97.
[101] Substance Abuse and Mental Health Services Administration. The NSUDH report: substance use, abuse, and dependence among youths who have been in a jail or a detention center. Rockville, MD: Substance Abuse and Mental Health Services Administration, Office of Applied Studies; 2004.
[102] CDC. Unintentional poisoning deaths—United States, 1999–2004. *MMWR* 2007;56:93–6.
[103] Reardon DC, Coleman PK, Cougle JR. Substance use associated with unintended pregnancy outcomes in the National Longitudinal Survey of Youth. *Am. J. Drug Alcohol. Abuse* 2004;30:369–83.
[104] Substance Abuse and Mental Health Services Administration. The NHSDA report: academic performance and youth substance use. Rockville, MD: Substance Abuse and Mental Health Services Administration, Office of Applied Studies; 2002.
[105] Kessler RC, Avenevoli S, Costello EJ, et al. Prevalence, persistence, and sociodemographic correlates of DSM-IV disorders in the National Comorbidity Survey Replication Adolescent Supplement. *Arch. Gen. Psychiatry 2012*;69:372–80.
[106] Shiffman S, Waters AJ, Hickcox M. The nicotine dependence syndrome scale: a multidimensional measure of nicotine dependence. *Nicotine Tob. Res*. 2004;6:327–48.
[107] Fagerstrom KO. Measuring degree of physical dependence to tobacco smoking with reference to individualization of treatment. *Addict Behav.* 1978;3:235–41.
[108] Heatherton TF, Kozlowski LT, Frecker RC, Fagerstrom KO. The Fagerstrom test for nicotine dependence: a revision of the Fagerstrom Tolerance Questionnaire. *Br. J. Addict.* 1991;86:1119–27.
[109] Bitsko RH, Danielson M, King M, Visser SN, Scahill L, Perou R. Health care needs of children with Tourette syndrome. *J. Child Neurol.* Published online November 8, 2012.
[110] Debes N, Hjalgrim H, Skov L. The presence of attention-deficit hyperactivity disorder (ADHD) and obsessive-compulsive disorder worsen psychosocial and educational problems in Tourette syndrome. *J. Child Neurol.* 2010;24.
[111] Robinson LR, Bitsko RH, Schieve LA, Visser SN. Tourette syndrome, parenting aggravation, and the contribution of co-occurring conditions

among a nationally representative sample. *Disabil. Health J.* 2013;6:26–35.

[112] CDC. Prevalence of diagnosed Tourette syndrome in persons aged 6–17 years—United States, 2007. MMWR 2009;58:581–5.

[113] Khalifa N, von Knorring A-L. Prevalence of tic disorders and Tourette syndrome in a Swedish school population. *Dev. Med. Child Neurol.* 2003;45:315–9.

[114] Scahill L, Williams S, Schwab-Stone M, Applegate JO, Leckman JF. Tic disorders and disruptive behavior in a community sample. *Adv. Neurol.* 2006;99:184–90.

[115] Stefanoff P, Wolanczyk T, Gawrys AS, et al. Prevalence of tic disorders among schoolchildren in Warsaw, Poland. *Eur. Child Adolesc. Psychiatry* 2008;17:171–8.

[116] CDC. Self-reported frequent mental distress among adults—United States, 1993–1996 MMWR 1998;47:325–31.

[117] CDC. Measuring healthy days: population assessment of measuring health-related quality of life. Atlanta, GA: CDC; 2000.

[118] Moriarty DG, Zack MM, Kobau R. The Centers for Disease Control and Prevention's Healthy Days Measures—population tracking of perceived physical and mental health over time. *Health Qual. Life Outcomes* 2003;1:37.

[119] Crosby AE, Ortega L, Melanson C. Self-directed violence surveillance: uniform definitions and recommended data elements, version 1.0. Atlanta, GA: CDC; 2011.

[120] US Department of Health and Human Services. National strategy for suicide prevention: goals and objectives for action. Washington, DC: Office of the Surgeon General and National Action Alliance for Suicide Prevention; 2012.

[121] US Public Health Service. The Surgeon General's call to action to prevent suicide Washington, DC: *US Department of Health and Human Services*; 1999

[122] Akinbami LJ, Liu X, Pastor PN, Reuben CA. Attention deficit hyperactivity disorder among children aged 5–17 years in the United States, 1998–2009. Data brief. Hyattsville, MD: *National Center for Health Statistics*; 2011.

[123] 123 CDC. Increasing prevalence of parent-reported attention-deficit/ hyperactivity disorder among children—United States, 2003 and 2007. *MMWR* 2010;59:1439–43.

[124] Healthcare Cost and Utilization Project statistical briefs chronological. Most frequent conditions in U.S. hospitals. Rockville, MD: Agency for Healthcare Research and Quality; 2013.

[125] Moreno C, Laje G, Blanco C, Jiang H, Schmidt AB, Olfson M. National trends in the outpatient diagnosis and treatment of bipolar disorder in youth. *Arch. Gen. Psychiatry* 2007;64:1032–9.

[126] Pastor PN, Reuben CA. Diagnosed attention deficit hyperactivity disorder and learning disability: United States, 2004–2006. *Vital Health Stat.* 10 2008; (237):1–14.

[127] Kogan MD, Blumberg SJ, Schieve LA, et al. Prevalence of parent-reported diagnosis of autism spectrum disorder among children in the U.S., 2007. *Pediatrics* 2009;124:1395–403.

[128] American Psychiatric Association. DSM-5: The future of psychiatric diagnosis. Arlington, VA: American Psychiatric Association; 2012. Available at http://www.dsm5.org/Pages/Default.aspx.

[129] Comer JS, Pincus DB, Hofmann SG. Generalized anxiety disorder and the proposed associated symptoms criterion change for DSM-5 in a treatment-seeking sample of anxious youth. *Depress Anxiety* 2012; 29:994–1003.

[130] Mahjouri S, Lord CE. What the DSM-5 portends for research, diagnosis, and treatment of autism spectrum disorders. *Curr. Psychiatry Rep.* 2012;14:739–47.

[131] Sibley MH, Waxmonsky JG, Robb JA, Pelham WE. Implications of changes for the field: ADHD. *J. Learn. Disabil.* 2013;46:34–42.

[132] Wakefield JC. DSM-5: proposed changes to depressive disorders. *Curr. Med. Res. Opin.* 2012;28:335–45.

[133] Walkup JT, Ferrão Y, Leckman JF, Stein DJ, Singer HS. Tic disorders: some key issues for DSM-V. *Depress Anxiety* 2010;27:600–10.

[134] Paul Wellstone and Pete Domenici Mental Health Parity and Addiction Equity Act of 2008, Pub. L. No. 110–343, 122; Stat. 3765 (October 3, 2008).

[135] Patient Protection and Affordable Care Act. Health-related portions of the Health Care and Education Reconciliation Act, Pub. L. 111–152, 124; Stat. 1029 (March 30, 2010).

[136] American Academy of Child and Adolescent Psychiatry Committee on Health Care Access and Economics and Task Force on Mental Health. Improving mental health services in primary care: reducing administrative and financial barriers to access and collaboration. *Pediatrics* 2009;123:1248–51.

[137] Aronen ET, Noam GG, Weinstein SR. Structured diagnostic interviews and clinicians' discharge diagnoses in hospitalized adolescents. *J. Am. Acad. Child Adolesc. Psychiatry* 1993;32:674–81.

[138] Jensen PS, Rubio-Stipec M, Canino G, et al. Parent and child contributions to diagnosis of mental disorder: are both informants always necessary? *J. Am. Acad. Child Adolesc. Psychiatry* 1999; 38:1569–79.

[139] Jewell J, Handwerk M, Almquist J, Lucas C. Comparing the validity of clinician-generated diagnosis of conduct disorder to the diagnostic interview schedule for children. *J. Clin. Child Adolesc. Psychol.* 2004; 33:536–46.

[140] McGrath AM, Handwerk ML, Armstrong KJ, Lucas CP, Friman PC. The validity of the ADHD section of the Diagnostic Interview Schedule for Children. *Behav. Modif.* 2004;28:349–74.

[141] Wolraich ML, McKeown RE, Visser SN, et al. The prevalence of attention-deficit/hyperactivity disorder: its diagnosis and treatment in four school districts across two states. *J. Atten. Disord.* Epub September 12, 2012. Available at http://jad.sagepub.com/content/early/2012/09/12/1087054712453169.long.

[142] Gochman P, Miller R, Rapoport JL. Childhood-onset schizophrenia: the challenge of diagnosis. *Curr. Psychiatry Rep.* 2011;13:321–2.

[143] Estimation methodology for children with a serious emotional disturbance (SED). *Federal Register* 1997; October 6 ed:52139-45.

[144] Burns BJ, Costello EJ, Angold A, et al. Children's mental health service use across service sectors. *Health Aff.* (Millwood) 1995;14:147–59.

[145] Comer JS, Olfson M, Mojtabai R. National trends in child and adolescent psychotropic polypharmacy in office-based practice, 1996–2007. *J. Am. Acad. Child Adolesc. Psychiatry* 2010;49:1001–10.

[146] Egger HL, Angold A. Common emotional and behavioral disorders in preschool children: presentation, nosology, and epidemiology. *J. Child Psychol. Psychiatry* 2006;47:313–37.

[147] Olfson M, Blanco C, Liu SM, Wang S, Correll CU. National trends in the office-based treatment of children, adolescents, and adults with antipsychotics. *Arch. Gen. Psychiatry* 2012;69:1247–56.

[148] Zito JM, Safer DJ, de Jong-van den Berg LT, et al. A three-country comparison of psychotropic medication prevalence in youth. Child *Adolesc. Psychiatry Ment. Health* 2008;2:26.

[149] Zito JM, Safer DJ, dosReis S, Gardner JF, Boles M, Lynch F. Trends in the prescribing of psychotropic medications to preschoolers. *JAMA* 2000;283:1025–30.

[150] 150 Mercy JA, Rosenberg ML, Powell KE, Broome CV, Roper WL. Public health policy for preventing violence. *Health Aff.* (Millwood) 1993;12:7–29.

In: Mental Health of Children and Adults … ISBN: 978-1-62808-626-3
Editor: George H. Jackson

Chapter 2

MENTAL ILLNESS SURVEILLANCE AMONG ADULTS IN THE UNITED STATES*

William C. Reeves, Tara W. Strine, Laura A. Pratt, William Thompson, Indu Ahluwalia, Satvinder S. Dhingra, Lela R. McKnight-Eily, Leslie Harrison, Denise V. D'Angelo, Letitia Williams, Brian Morrow, Deborah Gould and Marc A. Safran

SUMMARY

Mental illnesses account for a larger proportion of disability in developed countries than any other group of illnesses, including cancer and heart disease. In 2004, an estimated 25% of adults in the United States reported having a mental illness in the previous year. The economic cost of mental illness in the United States is substantial, approximately $300 billion in 2002. Population surveys and surveys of health-care use measure the occurrence of mental illness, associated risk behaviors (e.g., alcohol and drug abuse) and chronic conditions, and use of mental health–related care and clinical services. Population-based surveys and surveillance systems provide much of the evidence needed to guide effective mental health promotion, mental illness prevention, and treatment programs.

* This Morbidity and Mortality Weekly Report, Vol. 60, Supplement, was released by the Centers for Disease Control and Prevention on September 2, 2011.

This report summarizes data from selected CDC surveillance systems that measure the prevalence and impact of mental illness in the U.S. adult population. CDC surveillance systems provide several types of mental health information: estimates of the prevalence of diagnosed mental illness from self-report or recorded diagnosis, estimates of the prevalence of symptoms associated with mental illness, and estimates of the impact of mental illness on health and well-being. Data from the CDC 2005–2008 National Health and Nutrition Examination Survey indicate that 6.8% of adults had moderate to severe depression in the 2 weeks before completing the survey. State-specific data from the CDC 2006 Behavioral Risk Factor Surveillance System (BRFSS), the most recent BRFSS data available, indicate that the prevalence of moderate to severe depression was generally higher in southeastern states compared with other states. Two other CDC surveys on ambulatory care services, the National Ambulatory Medical Care Survey and the National Hospital Ambulatory Medical Care Survey, indicate that during 2007–2008, approximately 5% of ambulatory care visits involved patients with a diagnosis of a mental health disorder, and most of these were classified as depression, psychoses, or anxiety disorders.

Future surveillance should pay particular attention to changes in the prevalence of depression both nationwide and at the state and county levels. In addition, national and state-level mental illness surveillance should measure a wider range of psychiatric conditions and should include anxiety disorders. Many mental illnesses can be managed successfully, and increasing access to and use of mental health treatment services could substantially reduce the associated morbidity.

INTRODUCTION

Mental illness refers collectively to all diagnosable mental disorders and is characterized by sustained, abnormal alterations in thinking, mood, or behavior associated with distress and impaired functioning [1]. Mental illness is an important public health problem, both in its own right and because the condition is associated with other chronic diseases and their resulting morbidity and mortality. According to the World Health Organization (WHO), mental illnesses account for more disability in developed countries than any other group of illnesses, including cancer and heart disease [2]. Approximately one fourth of adults in the United States have a mental illness, and nearly half will develop at least one mental illness during their lifetime [3–5]. The most common mental illnesses in adults are anxiety and mood disorders [4]. The effects of mental illness range from minor disruptions in daily functioning to incapacitating personal, social, and occupational impairments and premature death (6–9). In 2002 and 2003, mental illness cost the United States an estimated $300 billion annually, which included approximately $193 billion from lost earnings and wages and $24 billion in disability benefits in 2002 [10] and $100 billion in health-care expenditures in 2003 [11].

Mental illness exacerbates morbidity from the multiple chronic diseases with which it is associated, including cardiovascular disease, diabetes, obesity, asthma, epilepsy, and cancer [12–16]. This increased morbidity is a result of lower use of medical care and treatment adherence for concurrent chronic diseases and higher risk for adverse health outcomes [17–20]. Rates for injuries, both intentional (e.g., homicide and suicide) and unintentional (e.g., motor vehicle), are 2–6 times higher among persons with a mental illness than in the overall population [21,22]. Mental illness also is associated with use of tobacco products and alcohol abuse [23].

This report summarizes data from selected CDC surveillance and information systems that measure mental illness and the associated effects in the U.S. adult population. The data presented include 1) the occurrence and associated effects of mental illness among adults in the United States as measured through selected CDC surveillance and information systems, 2) the CDC systems involved in the collection of mental illness data for adults and the associated public access databases, and 3) estimates from other studies and surveys, particularly those conducted by the Substance Abuse and Mental Health Services Administration (SAMHSA), compared with CDC system estimates.

BACKGROUND

Role of Surveillance in Reducing Morbidity and Mortality Associated with Mental Illness

Public health surveillance is the ongoing and systematic collection, analysis, interpretation, and dissemination of data used to develop public health interventions that reduce morbidity and mortality and improve health [24]. Surveillance for a particular condition might depend either on collection of new data or use of data obtained from existing health information systems (e.g., from vital statistics or public health surveys). Surveillance data have numerous uses in public health: 1) determination of the distribution and spread of disease, 2) estimation of the impact of a disease or injury, 3) generation of hypotheses and stimulation of research, 4) development of public health interventions, 5) description of the history of a health condition and the impact of treatments on outcomes, 6) evaluation of prevention and control measures, and 7) facilitation of program planning [25]. Because a single surveillance system typically cannot accomplish all of these tasks, use of multiple surveillance systems often provides a more complete assessment of a particular disease or condition.

Surveillance data are essential to the public health goals of reducing the incidence, prevalence, severity, and economic impact of mental illnesses. Public health officials, academicians, health-care providers, and advocacy groups need accurate and timely information on the prevalence and effects of mental illness to detect and characterize trends in mental illness prevalence and severity [26]; assess associations between mental illness and other chronic medical conditions (e.g., obesity, diabetes, heart disease, and alcohol and substance abuse); identify populations at high risk for mental illness and target interventions, treatment, and prevention measures; and provide outcome measures for evaluating mental illness interventions. For example, officials have used metal illness surveillance data to track trends in mental illness and psychological distress associated with exposure to military combat or large-scale disasters [27].

Diagnostic Classification of Mental Illness

Population surveys can be used to estimate accurately the prevalence of certain mental illness symptoms across populations, and by repeating surveys over time, they can be used to detect and characterize trends. Surveys generally cannot be used to diagnose mental disorders with the same level of specificity as an individual clinical examination conducted by an experienced psychiatrist or other mental health professional. Instead, they collect information on a range of subjective manifestations of alterations in thinking, mood, behavior, and associated distress that correspond with clinical disorders. Surveys collect this information using participant questionnaires that have been validated empirically to distinguish between persons with and without specific mental illnesses or general psychological distress. Estimates from these surveys vary according to the symptoms being collected and the way they correspond with various defined mental illnesses. Survey estimates usually are based on carefully defined patterns of symptoms. The most commonly used patterns correspond with diagnostic criteria agreed on by mental health professionals.

The symptom patterns used for surveys vary according to the classification of mental illness under study; changes in these classifications over time have increased the complexity of matching symptom patterns to specific illnesses. New classifications have been identified, and certain classifications have been removed. Even for relatively stable diagnostic categories (e.g., depression), subcategories and terminology have varied over time. For example, terms used to describe depression have included major and minor depression, psychotic depression, depression not otherwise specified, bipolar disorder, dysthymia, moderate to severe depression, and mild depression. However, the relationship among the disorders described by these different terms often is unclear. The American Psychiatric Association (APA) developed mental illness diagnostic categories based on symptoms observed by a health professional or reported by the patient; the Diagnostic and Statistical Manual of Mental Disorders, Fourth Edition, Text Revision (DSM-IV-TR) is the current version of this system (28). Another system, the WHO International Classification of Diseases, 10th Revision, Clinical Modification (ICD-10-CM), defines mental illness categories that are similar but not identical to those in the DSM-IV-TR (29). Previous DSM and ICD versions have not been completely congruent, and APA is developing a fifth edition of the DSM (DSM-V) that will coordinate better with future editions of ICD [30].

Methods for Measuring Prevalence and Public Health Impact of Mental Illness

Research Instruments

The Structured Clinical Interview for DSM Disorders (SCID) Research Version [31] is considered to be the standard among psychiatric research instruments based on DSM-IV-TR criteria; however, SCID takes 30–60 minutes and must be conducted by a trained mental health professional. Another instrument, the Composite International Diagnostic Interview (CIDI), was developed by WHO and is based on ICD-10 mental illness criteria. CIDI also is intended for use in epidemiological, clinical, and research studies. CIDI is lengthy, like SCID, but may be administered by trained lay interviewers

[32]. SCID and CIDI identify overlapping but not necessarily identical populations because they are based on different classification systems.

Screening Instruments

Large surveys that focus on a wide range of health topics typically can include only a limited number of mental health questions and often rely on SCID- or CIDI-validated screening instruments to provide indicators of psychiatric-related symptoms; in some cases, statistical models are used to predict the likelihood of specific mental illness in the respondent based on rating scales. Several standardized and validated screening instruments can be used to identify persons with mental illnesses such as depression and psychological distress, with varying degrees of diagnostic sensitivity and specificity [33–35]. CDC surveys use these screening instruments, as well as other standardized questions, to assess mental illness and other measures, such as impaired quality of life (e.g., mentally unhealthy days) and health-related disability associated with mental illness.

Depression (Patient Health Questionnaire-8 and Patient Health Questionnaire-9)

Depression is a major focus of population surveys of mental illness. To meet the DSM-IV-TR definition of major depressive disorder, a person must have either a depressed mood or a loss of interest or pleasure in daily activities consistently for at least 2 weeks. This mood must represent a change from the person's normal mood; social, occupational, educational, or other important functioning also must be impaired by the change in mood. Under the DSM-IV-TR, a depressed mood that is caused by substances (e.g., drugs, alcohol, or medications) or that is part of a general medical condition is not considered to be major depressive disorder [28].

One of the most widely used and validated instruments for measuring depression in population surveys is the nine-item Patient Health Questionnaire (PHQ-9). The PHQ-9 screens for the presence of the nine DSM-IV-TR criteria for acute and clinically significant depressive disorders [36]. A PHQ-9 score of ≥ 10 has high sensitivity (88%) and specificity (88%) when validated against SCID [37] and effectively detects depressive symptoms among persons of various races and ethnicities [38,39]. The PHQ-9 has been used as a self-administered module in many clinical studies and telephone-administered surveys [38,40–43]. Other telephone surveys have used a slightly shorter instrument, the eight-item Patient Health Questionnaire (PHQ-8), which omits the PHQ-9 question concerning suicidal or self-injurious ideation because survey administrators might not be able to offer appropriate follow-up interventions. Omitting this question in population-based surveys has only a minor effect on the usefulness of PHQ as a screen for depression [36].

The standard PHQ-8 and PHQ-9 have the following primary question: "Over the last 2 weeks, how often have you been bothered by any of the following problems?" The following problems are listed: 1) little interest or pleasure in doing things; 2) feeling down, depressed, or hopeless; 3) trouble falling/staying asleep, sleeping too much; 4) feeling tired or having little energy; 5) poor appetite or overeating; 6) feeling bad about yourself or that you are a failure or have let yourself or your family down; 7) trouble concentrating on things, such as reading the newspaper or watching television; 8) moving or speaking so slowly that other people could have noticed, or the opposite — being so fidgety or restless that you have been moving around a lot more than usual; and 9) (PHQ-9 only) thoughts that you would be better off dead or of hurting yourself in some way. Response categories are "not at all," "several days," "more than half the days," and "nearly every day."

PHQ-8 and PHQ-9 answers are scored using one of two algorithms, and the scores are used to assign depression categories. One algorithm is based on the DSM-IV and categorizes depressed respondents as having a major depressive disorder or other depression. The other algorithm categorizes respondents according to the severity of depressive symptoms (i.e., no significant depressive symptoms or mild, moderate, moderately severe, or severe depressive symptoms) [36,37].

Psychological Distress (Kessler-6 Psychological Distress Scale)

Surveys use the Kessler-6 psychological distress scale to screen for psychological distress experienced by persons with anxiety and mood disorders [44]. The Kessler-6 scale asks respondents about the frequency with which they have experienced six manifestations of psychological distress, which include feeling 1) nervous, 2) hopeless, 3) restless or fidgety, 4) so sad or depressed that nothing could cheer the respondent up, 5) that everything is an effort, and 6) worthless. Responses are "all of the time," "most of the time," "some of the time," "a little of the time," and "none of the time." Scoring of individual items is based on a 4-point scale according to increased frequency of the problem, yielding a total six-item score ranging from 0–24. A score of ≥13 indicates serious psychological distress [45]. Serious psychological distress as defined by the Kessler-6 score is highly associated with anxiety disorders and depression but does not identify a specific mental illness [44].

Mentally Unhealthy Days

Health-related quality of life (HRQOL) is a multidimensional concept that includes physical, mental, emotional, and social domains and reflects perceived physical and mental health [46,47]. HRQOL often is used to characterize certain aspects of disease impact, disability, and injury and to identify unmet health needs and disparities among various sociodemographic populations [48]. A core set of four questions (i.e., the Healthy Days Core Module, or HRQOL-4) has been standardized and validated for public health survey purposes. HRQOL-4 asks respondents about self-rated general health, physical health, mental health, and activity limitations resulting from poor physical or mental health during the previous 30 days [48]. One indicator often used to measure HRQOL is the number of mentally unhealthy days experienced by a person. Typically, the question asks: "Now thinking about your mental health, which includes stress, depression, and problems with emotions, for how many days during the past 30 days was your mental health not good?" Respondents who report ≥14 mentally unhealthy days over the past month are defined as having frequent mental distress. The mentally unhealthy days question has acceptable criterion validity and test-retest reliability [48–50]. In a large prospective study, this question predicted 1-month and 12-month physician visits, hospitalizations, and mortality outcomes [51].

Health-Care Surveys

Data from health-care providers and insurers provide an additional important source of information on the prevalence of mental illness in the United States. Coding systems used by hospitals and medical providers for billing purposes typically use the ICD-9 coding system, which, as mentioned previously, is not completely congruent with the DSM-IV-TR. In addition, mental health professionals generally use the DSM-IV-TR nomenclature, whereas primary care providers use other terminology. In practice, regardless of the diagnostic system used, diagnoses vary according to the training of the coder, local practice, availability of treatment resources, and reimbursement codes.

CDC Surveillance Systems and Surveys that Measure Prevalence and Impact of Mental Illness

CDC systems for measuring the prevalence and impact of mental illness in the U.S. adult population fall into two categories: 1) population surveys, which are used to estimate mental illness prevalence, and 2) national health-care surveys that include a diagnosed psychiatric condition based on ICD-9 codes, which are used to estimate outpatient visits and hospitalizations and reflect access to and use of health care by persons with mental illness (Table 1). Both of these systems provide public access data sets that allow researchers to address specific queries or conduct specific analyses. In combination with information from other studies and surveys, notably surveys conducted by SAMHSA, data from these CDC systems can be used to plan, implement, and evaluate mental illness prevention strategies and to explore ways to protect and promote mental health. Proper interpretation of mental health surveillance statistics requires an understanding of 1) the reason the data were collected (e.g., to identify prevalence or for program planning); 2) the survey population (e.g., representative of state or national population, sample frame, and time conducted); 3) survey methods (e.g., telephone vs. in-person interviews, record reviews or abstracts, and vital statistics); 4) questionnaires and questions used (e.g., standardization, validity, and reliability); 5) parameters measured (population prevalence and effects of the illness); and 6) appropriate analyses (adjustment and weighting for survey designs and response rates, rates, proportions, and continuous measures).

Population Surveys

BRFSS

BRFSS is a state-based telephone survey that was established in 1984.[1] BRFSS is the largest ongoing telephone health survey in the world, with approximately 450,000 adult interviews completed each year. BRFSS collects standardized, state-specific data concerning preventive health practices and risk behaviors associated with infectious diseases, chronic diseases, and injuries in the adult population. Data are collected in all 50 states, the District of Columbia, Puerto Rico, the U.S. Virgin Islands, and Guam. The large size of the survey permits calculation of state-specific estimates (and in some cases, substate estimates) and aggregated nationwide estimates. States use BRFSS data to identify emerging health problems, establish and track health objectives, and develop and evaluate public health policies and programs. For many states, BRFSS is the only source of timely, accurate, state-based data on health-related behaviors.

BRFSS interviews consist of three parts: 1) core questions asked in all states and territories (e.g., demographics, HRQOL, access to health care, disability, chronic conditions, and risk behaviors); 2) optional modules with questions on specific topics (for mental illness: the anxiety and depression module and the mental illness and stigma module); and 3) questions added by individual states. BRFSS data are directly weighted for the probability of selection of a telephone number, the number of adults in a household, and the number of landline telephone numbers that reach a household. Data are then stratified to adjust for nonresponse, to adjust for noncoverage of households without telephones, and to force the sum of the weighted frequencies to equal the adult population in each state.

Every year, the core BRFSS includes a question on number of mentally unhealthy days as a measure of HRQOL. States also may administer BRFSS optional modules (conducted through a collaboration between CDC and SAMHSA) that address other mental health topics in depth. In 2006, 2008, and 2010, an optional BRFSS module on anxiety and depression contained the PHQ-8, one question on lifetime diagnosis of anxiety, and one question on lifetime diagnosis of depression.

In 2007 and 2009, an optional BRFSS module on mental illness and stigma included the Kessler-6 scale (past 30 days), one question on activity limitations associated with a mental health condition or emotional problem, one question on treatment, and two questions on attitudes toward mental illness that might underlie stigma. Because certain individual states do not use these optional modules, BRFSS cannot provide national estimates of depression or psychological distress.

CDC provides public online access to the following summary statistics from various BRFSS modules:

- Prevalence and trends data: prevalence estimates for core variables by year and by state from 1995 to the present [2]
- Selected metropolitan/micropolitan area risk trends (SMART) city and county data: CDC information on all health risk data for metropolitan and micropolitan statistical areas (MMSAs) by year and category, with users able to generate reports that compare statistics by MMSA and to use SMART to produce charts that show state, MMSA, and county data for a limited set of health risk factors (2002–2008)[3,4]
- BRFSS maps: MMSA maps for many core variables (2002– present)[5] and annual BRFSS survey data and technical documentation so that researchers can conduct their own analyses
- Yearly state-based survey data sets and technical documentation (1984–present)[6]
- Yearly data sets and technical documentation for counties and MMSAs with ≥500 respondents (2002–present)[7]
- Yearly data and technical documentation for state and MMSA geographic information system data files (2002–present)[8]

National Health Interview Survey

The National Health Interview Survey (NHIS) is a continuous cross-sectional survey of the civilian U.S. household population. NHIS monitors the health of the U.S. population through the collection and analysis of data on a broad range of health topics.[9] Data are collected through an in-person household interview. The basic module, which remains largely unchanged from year to year, includes three components: a family core questionnaire, a sample adult core questionnaire, and a sample child core questionnaire. The family core collects information on everyone in the family and serves as the sampling frame for additional integrated surveys. This core includes information concerning household composition and sociodemographic characteristics, tracking information, information for linkage to administrative databases, indicators of health status, activity limitations, injuries, health insurance coverage, and access to and use of health-care services. One adult and one child (if any children aged <18 years are present) are selected randomly from each family, and information on each is collected with the sample adult core and sample child core questionnaires. Because certain health issues are different for adults and children, certain items on these two questionnaires differ; however, both collect basic data on health status, health-care services, and behavior. These sections of the survey yield the sample adult and the sample child data files.

NHIS uses a multistage area probability design to identify representative U.S. households. The sample is redesigned and redrawn approximately every 10 years to more accurately measure the changing population and to meet new survey objectives. NHIS oversamples blacks, Hispanics, and Asians (especially those aged ≥65 years) to allow for more precise estimation of health characteristics in these growing minority populations. The NHIS sample size (approximately 10,000) is not sufficient to provide reliable state-level estimates for most states. Although the database does not identify respondents' state of residence, state-level estimates can be produced for more populous states by requesting state identifiers through the CDC National Center for Health Statistics (NCHS) Research Data Centers.[10]

NHIS sample weights, which account for the differential probabilities of selection, nonresponse, and noncoverage, must be used for all analyses. Methods that incorporate the complex sample design and weights (e.g., Taylor series linearization) must be used to calculate appropriate standard errors.

Since 1997, NHIS has used the Kessler-6 scale (past 30 days) to identify serious psychological distress among adults. National rates for psychological distress by age, sex, and race are produced quarterly through the NHIS Early Release Program and are available online. In 2007, the NHIS included three questions on lifetime diagnoses: "Have you EVER been told by a doctor or other health professional that you had bipolar disorder? Schizophrenia? Mania or psychoses?"

National Health and Nutrition Examination Survey

The National Health and Nutrition Examination Survey (NHANES) is a continuous survey of the health and nutritional status of the U.S. civilian noninstitutionalized population.[11] Although NHANES uses a multistage probability household sampling design to obtain a nationally representative sample, the sample is not sufficient for state- or local-level analyses. NHANES sample weights, which account for the differential probabilities of selection, nonresponse, and noncoverage, must be used for all analyses. Survey participants complete an interview administered in their home and then are invited to participate in an examination conducted in a mobile examination center. This includes a private interview, a standardized physical examination, and collection of biological specimens for laboratory testing. NHANES collects data on the prevalence of 1) chronic diseases and conditions (including undiagnosed conditions detected through the examination or laboratory testing) and risk factors (e.g., obesity, smoking, serum cholesterol levels, hypertension, and diet and nutritional status), 2) vaccination status, 3) infectious disease prevalence, 4) health insurance, and 5) measures of environmental exposures. Other topics include hearing, vision, anemia, diabetes, cardiovascular disease, osteoporosis, oral health, pharmaceuticals and dietary supplements, physical fitness, HRQOL, and health-care use. In the private mobile examination center interview, NHANES uses the PHQ-9 to measure depression, and since 2000, this NHANES interview also has included the question on number of mentally unhealthy days. The examination and laboratory data collected allow researchers to examine the relationships between depression and health variables not available on other national surveys.

Pregnancy Risk Assessment Monitoring System

The Pregnancy Risk Assessment Monitoring System (PRAMS) was established in 1987 and is a state-based, cross-sectional survey of women who have recently delivered a live-born infant. PRAMS provides population-based data that can be used to develop maternal and infant health programs and policies.[12] The survey uses a mixed-mode data collection method. Each month, randomly selected women who have delivered a live-born infant are requested to complete a mail questionnaire; follow-up with nonresponders occurs by phone. Data are collected in 37 states and New York City, representing approximately 75% of the births in the United States. Data are weighted to adjust for survey design, nonresponse, and noncoverage.

PRAMS collects information on maternal behaviors, attitudes, and experiences before, during, and after pregnancy. Survey responses are linked to birth certificate data. The questionnaire includes core questions asked of all participants in all states, optional standard questions pretested by CDC, and state-developed questions. PRAMS provides estimates of postpartum depression by using two questions similar to those included in the PHQ-8: 1) "Since your new baby was born, how often have you felt down, depressed, or hopeless?" and 2) "Since your new baby was born, how often have you had little interest in doing things?" Possible responses are "never," "rarely," "sometimes," "often," and "always." Women who answer "often" or "always" to either question or both questions are categorized as having postpartum depression.

CDC provides access to PRAMS data electronically through CPONDER (CDC's PRAMS On-line Data for Epidemiologic Research).[13] CPONDER provides access to prevalence estimates by state and by year (2000–2008). In addition, CPONDER indexes 54 variables by topic for selection as the outcome variable in cross-tabular analyses. Twelve control variables may be used to stratify these outcomes in an analysis. Analyses may include a single state and all available years or all available states and a single year.

NATIONAL HEALTH-CARE SURVEYS

CDC conducts surveys of health-care providers, and the data from these surveys complement data from the population-based surveys to provide a more complete representation of the occurrence of mental illness in the United States. For the health-care surveys, CDC collects data from a sample of organizations that provide health care (e.g., nursing homes, inpatient hospitals, or physician offices). The data can be used to examine factors that influence use of health-care resources, quality of health care, and disparities in health-care services in population subgroups. In addition, because the surveys collect core information from a sample of providers that remains relatively stable over time, trends in the types of care delivered in each setting can be monitored and examined in relation to the characteristics of providers, patients, and clinical management of patient care.

National Ambulatory Medical Care Survey

The National Ambulatory Medical Care Survey (NAMCS)[14] collects information on the use of ambulatory care services in the United States. NAMCS uses a multistage probability sample of visits to office-based physicians and health-care providers in community health centers and collects data on provider characteristics. Sample data are weighted to produce national estimates that describe the provision and use of ambulatory medical care services in the United States. Public use data files are released annually and include a visit statistical weight and (since 2005) a physician statistical weight. Information on mental health and mental illness available from NAMCS includes reasons for visit, physician diagnosis, medications, treatment, referrals, and one item on comorbid depression. Physician diagnoses are recorded as written by the physician (text or ICD-9 codes). Nosologists convert text to ICD-9 codes for the data files.

National Hospital Ambulatory Medical Care Survey

The National Hospital Ambulatory Medical Care Survey (NHAMCS)[14] collects data on the use of ambulatory care services in hospital emergency and outpatient departments. NHAMCS involves a multistage probability sample of visits to the emergency and outpatient departments of noninstitutional, general, and short-stay hospitals in the United States.

Federal, military, and U.S. Department of Veterans Affairs hospitals are not included. Data collected from outpatient departments are similar to those collected by NAMCS. Data from emergency department visits are slightly different from the outpatient department data and include whether the patient was admitted to a mental health unit or transferred to a psychiatric hospital. Sample data are weighted to produce national estimates. Public-use data files are released annually.

National Hospital Discharge Survey

The National Hospital Discharge Survey (NHDS)[15] obtains national-level information on characteristics of inpatients discharged from nonfederal, short-stay (<30 days) hospitals in the United States. Only hospitals with an average length of stay of <30 days, general hospitals, and children's general hospitals are included in the survey. Psychiatric hospitals with an average length of stay of <30 days are eligible. NHDS does not include federal, military, U.S. Department of Veterans Affairs hospitals, prison hospitals, or hospitals with fewer than six beds.

Hospitals are selected by using a three-stage stratified design. Patient information collected includes demographics, length of stay, diagnoses, and procedures. Hospital characteristics collected include region, ownership, and number of beds. NHDS sample statistical weights account for nonresponse and must be used for all analyses. Methods that incorporate the complex sample design and weights, such as Taylor series linearization, must be used to calculate appropriate standard errors.

National Nursing Home Survey

The National Nursing Home Survey (NNHS)[16] is a continuous series of national sample surveys of nursing homes and their residents and staff members. NNHS provides information on nursing homes from the perspectives of the provider and recipient of services. Data on facilities include characteristics such as number of beds, ownership, affiliation, Medicare and Medicaid certification, specialty units, services offered, number and characteristics of staff, expenses, and charges. Data on current residents include demographic characteristics, health status, up to 16 current diagnoses, level of assistance needed with activities of daily living, vision and hearing impairment, continence, services received, and sources of payment. The survey uses a stratified two-stage probability design. The first stage is the selection of facilities, and the second stage is selection of residents.

Findings from CDC Surveillance Systems and Surveys

Through the surveys and surveillance systems described in this report, CDC provides prevalence estimates on current depression, postpartum depression, psychological distress, number of mentally unhealthy days, and lifetime diagnosis of depression, anxiety, bipolar disorder, and schizophrenia in the U.S. adult population. CDC health-care surveys provide health services information about physician, hospital outpatient, and emergency department visits related to mental illness. All of these CDC systems can provide data for national-level (or nationwide) estimates by sex, age, race, and ethnicity. BRFSS and PRAMS data also can be used for state-level estimates.

Population Surveys

Current Depression

Two CDC surveillance systems provide estimates for current depression: NHANES (national estimates) and BRFSS (state estimates). These systems use the PHQ-9 (NHANES) or PHQ-8 (BRFSS) to estimate the occurrence of depression in the last 2 weeks. For example, using continuously collected data from 2005–2008 (the most recent data available), results from NHANES indicate that 6.8% of U.S. adults had depression (measured by the PHQ-9) during the 2 weeks before the survey (Table 2).

Results from BRFSS for current depression (measured by the PHQ-8) vary according to the year conducted because in different years, a varying number of states might have administered the optional modules containing the mental illness–related questions. Results from 2006 (in 38 states, the District of Columbia, Puerto Rico, and the U.S. Virgin Islands) using the PHQ-8 indicate that approximately 8.7% of respondents had current depression. Results from 2008 in 16 states using the optional BRFSS anxiety and depression module indicate that 8.2% had current depression. Prevalence estimates were higher among women and non-Hispanic blacks compared with other groups (Table 3).

Using the PHQ-8 algorithm for major depressive disorder (*36*), the 2006 BRFSS prevalence estimate of major depression during the previous 2 weeks was 3.5% (95% confidence interval [CI]: 3.3–3.7) and in 2008 was 3.0% (95% CI: 2.8–3.3). BRFSS state-specific prevalence estimates for depression in 2006 and 2008 show marked variations from state to state, with prevalences ranging from 4.3% in North Dakota to 13.7% in Mississippi and West Virginia (Table 4). The prevalence of depression was generally highest in the southeastern states (Figure 1).

Postpartum Depression

During 2004–2008, a total of 14.5% of PRAMS respondents reported symptoms of postpartum depression (i.e., answered "often" or "always" to either or both of the following questions): 1) "Since your new baby was born, how often have you felt down, depressed, or hopeless?" and 2) "Since your new baby was born, how often have you had little interest in doing things?") (Table 5).

The prevalence of postpartum depression varied by age, ranging from 10.3% among women aged 30–39 years to 23.3% among women aged ≤19 years. Prevalence also varied by race/ethnicity: 16.8% among Hispanic women, 11.9% among non-Hispanic white women, and 21.5% among non-Hispanic black women.

Among 22 states, the prevalence of postpartum depression ranged from 9.8% in Minnesota to 21.3% in Tennessee (Table 6).

Psychological Distress

Both NHIS and optional modules of BRFSS use the Kessler-6 scale to identify persons who experienced psychological distress during the 30 days before the survey. NHIS data indicate that in 2009, 3.2% of respondents experienced serious psychological distress (Table 7). BRFSS included the Kessler-6 in the optional mental illness and stigma module during 2007 (administered in 35 states, the District of Columbia, and Puerto Rico) and 2009 (16 states). Among participating states, prevalence estimates were similar in 2007 (4.0%) and 2009 (3.9%) (Table 8). These BRFSS estimates are higher than NHIS estimates, which might be a result of the limited geographical coverage of BRFSS, differences in survey design and methods, question placement, and context. As in NHIS, women were more likely to have serious psychological distress than men, and rates were highest among adults aged 45–54 years and non-Hispanic blacks. BRFSS data for state-specific prevalences of serious psychological distress during 2007 and 2009 indicate that, like depression, prevalence varied among states, ranging from 1.9% in Utah to 9.4% in Tennessee (Table 9). The prevalence of serious psychological distress was generally highest in the southeastern states (Figure 2).

Mentally Unhealthy Days

The question on number of mentally unhealthy days is included in the BRFSS core questionnaire; therefore, data are available for every year for all states and territories. Nationwide, for 2009, adults aged ≥18 years reported an average of 3.5 mentally unhealthy days during the past 30 days (Table 10). Among states, in 2009, the median number of mentally unhealthy days was 3.4, and the 25th and 75th quartiles were 3.1 and 3.7 days, respectively (Table 11). The mean number of mentally unhealthy days was highest in the southeastern states (Figure 3).

Lifetime Diagnosis of Mental Illness

The BRFSS optional anxiety and depression module includes questions on whether respondents have received a diagnosis of depression or anxiety disorder in their lifetime. Although the number of participating states varied between the 2 years in which the module was administered, rates of reported lifetime diagnosis of depression were similar in 2006 (15.7%) and 2008 (16.1%) (Tables 12 and 13). The prevalence of lifetime diagnosis of anxiety disorders was slightly lower, with 11.3% in 2006 and 12.3% in 2008 (Tables 14 and 15).

In 2007, NHIS included a question for all respondents on lifetime diagnosis of bipolar disorder and schizophrenia; 1.7% of participants had received a diagnosis of bipolar disorder, and 0.6% had received a diagnosis of schizophrenia (Table 16).

National Health-Care Surveys

NAMCS and NHAMCS

During 2007–2008, an estimated 47.8 million ambulatory care visits were made by patients with primary mental health diagnoses, which constituted approximately 5% of all ambulatory care visits made in the United States during those 2 years (Tables 17 and 18). Women made 29.4 million of the visits, compared with 18.5 million for men.

Of all mental illness–related visits, the greatest proportion of visits (31%) were made by patients with any depressive disorder, followed by 23% of visits among those with schizophrenia and other psychotic disorders. The proportion of visits related to alcohol and drug use that occurred in emergency and outpatient departments was higher than the proportion of visits for other mental illness diagnoses.

NHDS

Among patients discharged from nonfederal, short-stay hospitals, mental illness was a primary diagnosis for 97.9 discharged patients per 10,000 population among persons aged 18–64 years. The occurence decreased with age to 64.4 among those aged ≥65 years (Table 19). Mood disorders were the most common primary mental illness discharge diagnosis, and the occurence decreased with age, with a range of 46.0 per 10,000 population among patients aged 18–44 years to 19.2 per 10,000 population among those aged ≥65 years. Alcohol and drug use disorders were the second most common diagnoses and also decreased with age. In contrast to rates for primary diagnoses, discharges rates among patients with mental illness listed as any of the diagnoses increased with age, ranging from 231.4 discharged patients per 10,000 population among those aged 18–44 years to 650.8 per 10,000 population among those aged >65 years (Table 20). As with primary diagnoses of mental illness, mood disorders were the most common diagnosis, followed by alcohol and drug use disorders.

NNHS

The prevalence of nursing home residents with a primary diagnosis of mental illness in 2004 increased with age, ranging from 18.7% among those aged 65–74 years to 23.5% among those aged ≥85 years (Table 21). Dementia and Alzheimer disease were the most common primary diagnoses among nursing home residents with a primary diagnosis of mental illness, and the prevalence of each increased with age.

Among nursing home residents with any diagnosis of mental illness (among any of 16 current diagnoses), mood disorders and dementia were the most common diagnoses among residents aged 65–74 years and 75–84 years (Table 22).

Among residents aged ≥85 years, dementia (41.0%) was the most common mental illness, followed by mood disorders (35.3%). In 2004, approximately two thirds of nursing home residents had a diagnosis of a mental illness, and approximately one third of these had a mood disorder.

Discussion

CDC national surveillance surveys such as NHANES and NHIS are important for developing national policies and tracking progress toward national health goals such as those described in *Healthy People 2010* and *Healthy People 2020.* Data from these surveys are useful for national planning and research.

Two state-based CDC surveys, BRFSS and PRAMS, can provide data at the state or substate levels that can be used for both national and state-level planning. For example, variations in BRFSS estimates for certain mental illnesses might help determine the focus of certain mental health services.

The prevalence of current depression varies substantially by state (from 4.3% in North Dakota to 13.7% in Mississippi and West Virginia), as does the prevalence of serious psychological distress (from 1.9% in Utah to 9.4% in Tennessee).

These variations might reflect regional differences, including demographic characteristics, socioeconomic conditions, availability of and access to health-care services, and patterns of reimbursement for mental health services, that would be useful in planning [52,53]. Southeastern states generally have the highest prevalence of depression, serious psychological distress, and mean number of mentally unhealthy days. This finding likely reflects, in part, sociodemographics, access to and use of health care, and the association between mental illness and certain chronic diseases such as obesity, diabetes, and cardiovascular disease [13,14]. For some states, BRFSS, PRAMS, and other state-based surveys have provided mental illness data that state and local authorities have used to identify the need for services at the local or regional level.

CDC surveys focus on depression, and they lack sufficient data on anxiety disorders. Anxiety disorders are as common in the population as depression and, like depression and severe psychological distress, can result in high levels of impairment.

Moreover, the pathophysiologic characteristics of anxiety disorders are similar to those of depression and often are associated with the same chronic medical conditions [54–5].

The National Epidemiologic Survey on Alcohol and Related Conditions (NESARC), conducted by the National Institute on Alcohol Abuse and Alcoholism, estimated that during 2001–2002, 14% of U.S. adults had an anxiety disorder (7%, specific phobia; 3%, social phobia; 2%, generalized anxiety disorder; and 1%, panic disorder) [23]. Estimates from the 2003 National Comorbidity Survey Replication (NCS-R) were similar, indicating that 18% of adults had an anxiety disorder (9%, specific phobia; 7%, social phobia; 4%, posttraumatic stress disorder; and 3%, panic disorder); 56% of the disorders identified were categorized as serious or moderate [5]. Several standardized and validated scales can be used in telephone and in-person interviews to identify and classify anxiety disorders [57,58]. Better documentation of the impact of anxiety disorders might help guide national public health policy.

At the state and local levels, documenting the prevalence and impact of anxiety disorders might help ascertain the need for additional public health services for these disorders. Although CDC surveys and information systems have provided important information on the prevalence of mental illness, none of them was designed solely to monitor mental illness.

They are general surveillance tools that have added components on mental illness gradually over time as recognition of the importance of mental illness in public health has increased.

For example, NHANES and NHIS are national CDC surveys designed to monitor the entire range of public health diseases and conditions and can include only a limited number of questions concerning mental illness. Likewise, the state-based CDC BRFSS is designed to provide state and local estimates on a wide range of health behaviors. BRFSS mental illness questions are primarily contained in two small mental illness modules that are optional for states and are not included on the core BRFSS questionnaire administered by all states.

States may choose to administer the optional modules, but not all states do so because of financial constraints, competing state surveillance priorities, and limitations in the length of time respondents are willing to spend completing a telephone survey.

The willingness of the states to administer optional modules is affected by the rapid rise in the proportion of households that no longer contain a landline telephone [59].

Survey calls to cell phone numbers are limited to BRFSS core questions and do not include the optional survey modules, partly because cell phone respondents are not willing to spend as much time completing BRFSS questions as respondents using landline telephones. Recognizing that the number of households with landline telephones will continue to decrease, CDC is exploring additional methods to obtain a valid sample for mental illness questions in BRFSS. Increasingly, physicians and others who treat mental illness, as well as public health experts, are recognizing the substantial overlap between mental illness and diseases traditionally considered to be matters of public health concern.

The ability of certain mental illnesses to exacerbate morbidity from several chronic diseases is well-established. Recent studies have explored the causal pathways from mental illness to certain chronic diseases [60,61], highlighting the need for more accurate and timely information on the epidemiology of mental illness in the United States.

Future mental illness surveillance surveys should measure both depression and anxiety disorders and include more detailed questions concerning their impact on quality of life, associated chronic medical conditions, and issues such as family violence, alcohol and substance abuse, and access to and use of health care.

For example, CDC is collaborating with SAMHSA and the Gulf Coast states to conduct surveillance of mental illness in coastal regions affected by the 2010 Deepwater Horizon oil spill. This targeted surveillance effort uses standardized questionnaires to identify the occurrence of anxiety disorders, depression, and psychological distress, as well as the effects of mental illness on and use of mental illness services by the Gulf Coast population.

Increased awareness of the value of mental illness surveillance is important, as is identification of gaps in the available CDC data and data from other sources.

The impact of psychological distress and depression is well-documented, and the risk factors and associated issues such as access to and use of health services have been identified. Therefore, increased emphasis should be placed on using this information to initiate public health action and on using surveillance to measure outcomes.

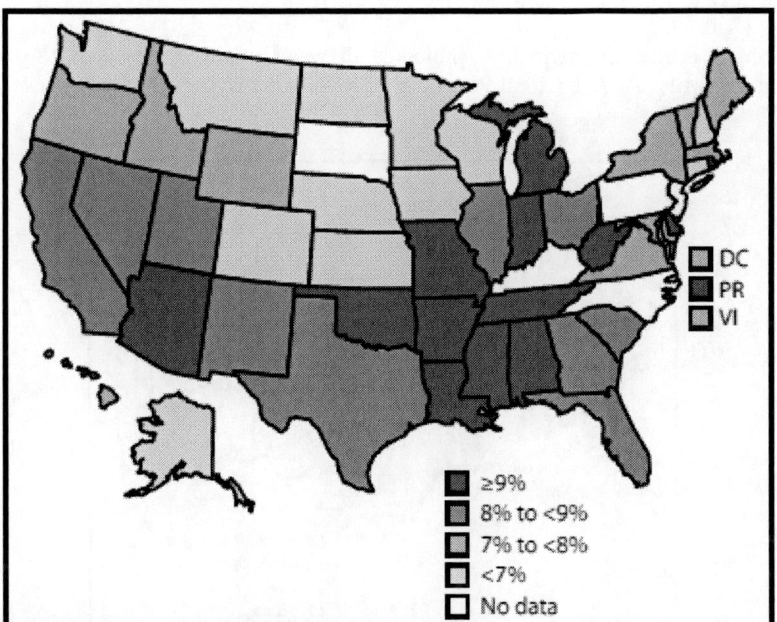

* Patient Health Questionnaire-8 severity score of >10.

† Quartiles based on point estimates (see Table 4).

§ For Arizona, Colorado, Idaho, Illinois, Massachusetts, New York, and Ohio, data are from 2008.

Figure 1. Prevalence of current depression* among adults aged ≥18 years, by state quartile† — Behavioral Risk Factor Surveillance System, United States, 2006§.

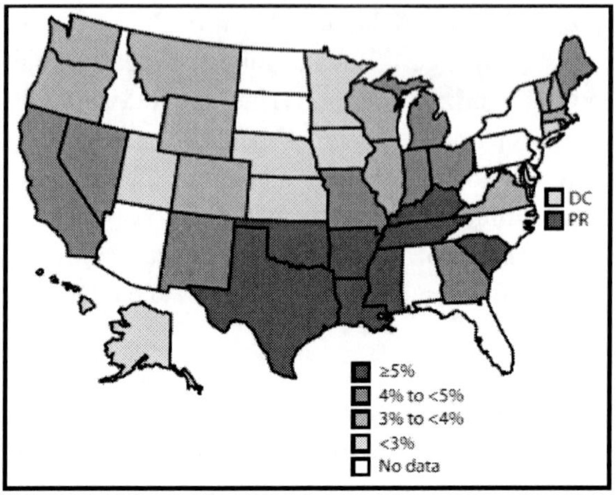

* Kessler-6 score of >13.

† For Tennessee and Utah, data are from 2009.

§ Quartiles based on point estimates (see Table 9).

Figure 2. Prevalence of serious psychological distress* among adults aged ≥18 years, by state quartile† — Behavioral Risk Factor Surveillance System, United States, 2007§.

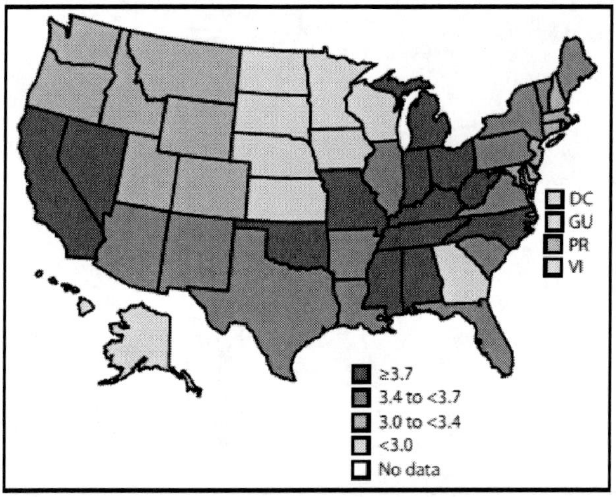

* Survey question: "Now thinking about your mental health, which includes stress, depression, and problems with emotions, for how many days during the last 30 days was your mental health not good?"

Figure 3. Mean number of mentally unhealthy days* during past 30 days among adults aged ≥18 years, by state quartile — Behavioral Risk Factor Surveillance System, United States, 2009.

Table 1. CDC surveys and surveillance systems that collect data on mental illness among adults

Name, website, and CDC sponsor	Description	Method of data collection	Survey topics	Mental health topics and questions	Population
Behavioral Risk Factor Surveillance System (BRFSS) http://www.cdc.gov/brfs shttp://www.cdc.gov/ brfss Public Health Surveillance Program Office	BRFSS is a state-based system of health surveys that collects information on health-risk behaviors, preventive health practices, and health-care access primarily related to chronic disease and injury. For many states, BRFSS is the only available source of timely, accurate data on health-related behaviors.	Telephone interviews	Heath-risk behaviors Preventive health practices Health-care access Health-related quality of life Mental illness screening Disability Violence	Anxiety and depression module (PHQ-8, lifetime diagnosis of anxiety and depression) Mental illness and stigma module (K-6, stigma, mental health treatment, and mental illness–related disability) Health-related quality of life (number of days in past 30 days respondent felt that mental health was not good, felt depressed, felt anxious, felt not getting enough sleep, and felt full of energy) Life satisfaction Social support Smoking, alcohol use, physical activity, and body mass index Health-care use and access Sexual and intimate partner violence	National sample of one person (aged ≥18 years)from each household Approximately 450,000 completed interviews, as of 2010

Table 1. (Continued)

Name, website, and CDC sponsor	Description	Method of data collection	Survey topics	Mental health topics and questions	Population
National Health Interview Survey (NHIS) http://www.cdc.gov/nchs/nhis.htmhttp://www.cdc.gov/nchs/nhis.htm National Center for Health Statistics	NHIS is a national survey on the health of the civilian noninstitutionalized U.S. population. The main objective of NHIS is to monitor the health of the U.S. population through the collection and analysis of data on a broad range of health topics.	In-person household interviews	Health status and limitations Health-care use Family resources Health insurance Health-care access Vaccination Injury Health behaviors Functioning Disability	Activity limitations from physical, mental, or emotional problems External causes and circumstances of injury Mental health-care use Mental health conditions and symptoms (in 2007 survey), including ADHD; schizophrenia; bipolar disorder; depression, anxiety, and emotional problems; dementia and senility; mental retardation; learning disabilities; and general distress symptoms Health-risk behaviors (including tobacco use and alcohol use) K-6 measure of serious psychological distress	Approximately 40,000 households per year, as of 2010 Oversample of blacks, Hispanics, Asians, and adults aged ≥65 years
National Health and Nutrition Examination Survey (NHANES)	NHANES is designed to assess the health and nutritional status of adults	In-person household interviews	Numerous diseases, medical conditions, and health indicators	Sleep disorders Alcohol and drug use Social and emotional support	Approximately 5,000 persons per year, as of 2008

Name, website, and CDC sponsor	Description	Method of data collection	Survey topics	Mental health topics and questions	Population
http://www.cdc.gov/nchs/nhanes.htmhttp://www.cdc.gov/nchs/nhanes.htm National Center for Health Statistics	and children in the United States. The survey combines interviews and physical examinations.	Physical examinations Laboratory tests Nutritional assessments DNA repository	Nutrition and nutritional disorders Environmental risk factors Health-care use Mental, behavioral, and emotional problems of children Weight and physical fitness Risk factors	Use of mental health-care professionals Activity limitations from poor physical or mental health PHQ-9 depression screening	Oversample of blacks, Mexican-Americans, adolescents, and adults aged ≥60 years
Pregnancy Risk Assessment Monitoring System (PRAMS) http://www.cdc.gov/pramshttp://www.cdc.gov/prams National Center for Chronic Disease Prevention and Health Promotion, Division of Reproductive Health	PRAMS is a surveillance project of CDC and state health departments. PRAMS collects state-specific, population-based data on maternal attitudes and experiences before, during, and shortly after pregnancy.	Mailed surveys with follow-up telephone interviews for nonresponders	Postpartum depressive symptoms Attitudes and feelings about most recent pregnancy Prenatal care Maternal alcohol and tobacco use HIV testing Health insurance coverage Physical abuse before and during pregnancy Pregnancy-related morbidity Infant health care	Whether health-care provider discussed with respondent healthy and risky pregnancy behaviors (including drinking alcohol and smoking during pregnancy) Maternal tobacco and alcohol use before, during, and after pregnancy Difficult or traumatic events before or during pregnancy Pregnancy intention, both of mother and of partner Whether respondent needed and received counseling for	Approximately 50,000 women with live-born infants per year, as of 2008

Table 1. (Continued)

Name, website, and CDC sponsor	Description	Method of data collection	Survey topics	Mental health topics and questions	Population
			Contraceptive use Breastfeeding practices Health-care provider advice	substance use or personal problems during or after pregnancy Interpersonal violence before and during pregnancy Injury control and prevention Social support and stress Infant sleeping behaviors Infant and maternal exposure to smoke Feelings, diagnosis, and treatment of postpartum depression, hopelessness, and anxiety	
National Ambulatory Medical Care Survey (NAMCS) http://www.cdc.gov/nchs/ahcd.htmhttp://www.cdc.gov/nchs/ahcd.htm National Center for Health Statistics	NAMCS is a national survey that collects data on the provision and use of ambulatory medical care services in the United States. Findings are based on a sample of visits to nonfederal, employed, office-based physicians who are primarily	Patient record forms completed by physicians and staff members or survey field representatives	Demographic characteristics of patients Expected payment sources Patients' principal complaints, symptoms, or other reasons for visit Physician diagnoses,	Current diagnosed mental health conditions Current depression Cause of injury (including intentional) Health education services ordered or provided at visit (including injury prevention, stress management, and tobacco use and exposure)	Office-based physicians andthen visits within the practices. In 2007, data were provided on 32,778 visits.

Name, website, and CDC sponsor	Description	Method of data collection	Survey topics	Mental health topics and questions	Population
	engaged in direct patient care.		diagnostic and screening services Medications Types of health-care providers seen during visit Disposition Causes of injury (if applicable)	Nonmedication treatment provided at visit (including psychotherapy and mental health counseling) Type of health-care providers patient visited or was referred to during visit (including providers of mental health services) Medications	
National Hospital Ambulatory Medical Care Survey (NHAMCS) http://www.cdc.gov/nchs/ahcd.htmhttp://www.cdc.gov/nchs/ahcd.htm National Center for Health Statistics	NHAMCS is designed to collect data on the use and provision of ambulatory care services in hospital emergency and outpatient departments. Findings are based on a national sample of visits to the emergency departments and outpatient departments of noninstitutional general and short-stay hospitals.	Patient record forms completed by hospital physicians and staff members	Demographic characteristics of patients Expected payment sources Patients' principal complaints, symptoms, or other reasons for visit Physician diagnoses, diagnostic and screening services Procedures (emergency department only) Medications Disposition Types of health- care	*Emergency department:* Patients' principal complaints, symptoms, or other reasons for visit Causes of injury (including intentional) Health-care provider diagnoses Medications Mental health providers seen during visit Transfer to psychiatric hospital Admission to mental health or detoxification unit *Outpatient department*: Current diagnosed mental	Nationally representative sample of 500 nonfederal short-stay (<30 days) hospitals

Table 1. (Continued)

Name, website, and CDC sponsor	Description	Method of data collection	Survey topics	Mental health topics and questions	Population
			providers seen during visit Causes of injury (if applicable)	health conditions Current depression Cause of injury (including intentional) Health education services ordered or provided at visit (including injury prevention, stress management, and tobacco use and exposure) Nonmedication treatment provided at visit (including psychotherapy and mental health counseling) Type of health-care providers patient visited or was referred to during visit (including providers of mental health services) Medications	
National Hospital Discharge Survey (NHDS) http://www.cdc.gov/nchs/nhds.htmhttp://www.c	NHDS is a national probability survey of characteristics of inpatients discharged from nonfederal short-stay	Medical record abstraction	Demographic characteristics of patients Expected sources of payment	Discharge diagnoses (up to seven) Surgical and diagnostic procedures (up to four)	Nationally representative sample of nonfederal short-stay hospitals and

Name, website, and CDC sponsor	Description	Method of data collection	Survey topics	Mental health topics and questions	Population
dc.gov/nchs/nhds.htm National Center for Health Statistics	hospitals in the United States.		Type and source of admission Disposition Discharge diagnoses (up to seven) Surgical and diagnostic procedures (up to four)		systematic samples of discharges within hospitals
National Nursing Home Survey (NNHS) http://www.cdc.gov/nchs/nnhs.htmhttp://www.cdc.gov/nchs/nnhs.htm National Center for Health Statistics	NNHS is a continuing series of national sample surveys of nursing homes and their residents and staff members.	Interviews with staff member best acquainted with resident medical records	Demographic characteristics of patients Admitting diagnosis Current diagnoses (up to 16) Health status Activities of daily living Vision and hearing Continence Pain assessment Behavior Mood Medications Falls Services received Sources of payment	Behavioral problems Depressed mood Medications Admitting diagnosis Current diagnoses (up to 16) Current assignment to specialty unit (i.e., dementia or behavioral health) Decision-making ability	Sample of nursing homes (that had at least three bedsand were either certified by Medicare or Medicaid or had a state license to operate as a nursing home) and then sample of residents within nursing homes

Abbreviations: ADHD = attention deficit hyperactivity disorder; HIV = human immunodeficiency virus; K-6 = Kessler-6; PHQ-8 = Patient Health Questionnaire-8; PHQ-9 = Patient Health Questionnaire-9.

Table 2. Prevalence of depression* among adults aged ≥18 years, by sociodemographic characteristics — National Health and Nutrition Examination Survey, United States, 2005–2008

Characteristic	No.	%	(95% CI)
Total	10,279	6.8	(5.8–7.8)
Sex Male	6,240	4.9	(3.9–5.9)
Female	6,397	8.4	(7.4–9.4)
Age group (yrs)			
18–39	4,093	6.2	(5.2–7.2)
40–59	2,992	8.4	(6.8–10.0)
>60	3,194	5.2	(4.0–6.4)
Race/Ethnicity Mexican-American	1,983	7.2	(5.6–8.8)
Black, non-Hispanic	2,273	9.7	(7.9–11.5)
White, non-Hispanic	4,882	6.2	(5.0–7.4)

Abbreviation: CI = confidence interval.

* Patient Health Questionnaire-9 score of >10.

Table 3. Prevalence of current depression* among adults aged ≥18 years, by sociodemographic characteristics and year — Behavioral Risk Factor Surveillance System, multiple states, 2006 and 2008

		2006†			2008§	
Characteristic	No.	%	(95% CI)	No.	%	(95% CI)
Total	198,678	8.7	(8.4–9.0)	85,004	8.2	(7.8–8.6)
Sex Male	76,288	6.8	(6.4–7.3)	32,243	6.6	(6.1–7.2)
Female	122,390	10.5	(10.1–10.9)	52,761	9.8	(9.2–10.3)
Age group (yrs)						

		2006†			2008§	
Characteristic	No.	%	(95% CI)	No.	%	(95% CI)
18–24	9,186	10.9	(9.7–12.2)	2,963	10.2	(8.5–12.2)
25–34	24,493	8.7	(8.0–9.4)	8,327	8.3	(7.3–9.4)
35–44	34,910	8.8	(8.2–9.4)	12,967	8.3	(7.5–9.3)
45–54	42,321	9.9	(9.3–10.5)	18,071	10.2	(9.4–11.1)
>55	86,396	6.9	(6.5–7.3)	42,071	6.1	(5.7–6.6)
Race/Ethnicity						
White, non-Hispanic	153,642	8.0	(7.7–8.3)	68,695	7.5	(7.1–7.9)
Black, non-Hispanic	15,819	11.0	(10.1–12.1)	4,837	12.7	(11.1–14.6)
Other, non-Hispanic¶	11,955	10.4	(9.3–11.7)	6,258	9.4	(7.9–11.2)
Hispanic	15,602	9.9	(8.9–11.0)	4,458	9.5	(7.9–11.3)

Abbreviation: CI = confidence interval.

* Patient Health Questionnaire-8 depression severity score of >10.

† Data from 38 states, District of Columbia, Puerto Rico, and U.S. Virgin Islands.

§ Data from 16 states.

¶ Asian, Native Hawaiian/Pacific Islander, American Indian/Alaska Native, other race, and multiple races.

Table 4. Prevalence of current depression* among adults aged ≥18 years, by state/area and year — Behavioral Risk Factor Surveillance System, United States, 2006 and 2008

		2006			2008	
State/Area	No.	%	(95% CI)	No.	%	(95% CI)
Alabama	2,758	12.5	(10.4–15.0)	—	—	—
Alaska	1,806	6.7	(5.4–8.2)	—	—	—

Table 4. (Continued)

		2006			2008	
State/Area	No.	%	(95% CI)	No.	%	(95% CI)
Arizona	—†	—	—	5,314	9.7	(8.0–11.7)
Arkansas	4,809	12.2	(11.0–13.4)	—	—	—
California	5,177	8.8	(7.8–9.9)	—	—	—
Colorado	—	—	—	5,093	7.0	(6.0–8.1)
Connecticut	4,109	5.9	(5.0–6.9)	—	—	—
Delaware	3,780	8.2	(6.9 – 9.6)	—	—	—
District of Columbia	3,485	7.9	(6.6–9.4)	—	—	—
Florida	9,298	8.9	(7.9–9.9)	—	—	—
Georgia	6,485	8.2	(7.3–9.2)	—	—	—
Hawaii	5,840	7.2	(6.3–8.1)	5,901	7.4	(6.5–8.5)
Idaho	—	—	—	4,570	7.6	(6.6–8.7)
Illinois	—	—	—	4,879	8.4	(7.4–9.6)
Indiana	5,746	9.6	(8.7–10.7)	—	—	—
Iowa	4,692	5.8	(5.0–6.7)	—	—	—
Kansas	3,797	6.9	(5.9–8.1)	3,783	8.6	(7.4–9.9)
Louisiana	5,774	9.5	(8.5–10.5)	5,388	9.3	(8.3–10.4)
Maine	3,605	7.4	(6.4–8.6)	3,724	7.8	(6.8–9.0)
Maryland	4,261	7.5	(6.3–8.8)			
Massachusetts	—	—	—	5,835	7.1	(6.2–8.2)
Michigan	5,077	10.5	(9.4–11.8)	—	—	—
Minnesota	4,119	6.2	(5.4–7.2)	—	—	—
Mississippi	5,225	13.0	(11.8–14.2)	6,387	13.7	(12.5–15.0)
Missouri	4,771	9.4	(8.3–10.7)	—	—	—

State/Area		2006			2008	
	No.	%	(95% CI)	No.	%	(95% CI)
Montana	5,262	6.7	(5.8–7.6)	—	—	—
Nebraska	3,516	5.6	(4.6–6.9)	4,840	8.5	(6.9–10.3)
Nevada	3,222	9.0	(7.5–10.7)	—	—	—
New Hampshire	5,230	6.8	(6.0–7.8)	—	—	—
New Mexico	5,745	9.3	(8.3–10.5)	—	—	—
New York	—	—	—	3,444	7.3	(6.3–8.4)
North Dakota	4,164	5.3	(4.4–6.2)	4,482	4.3	(3.6–5.1)
Ohio	—	—	—	5,797	9.2	(8.2–10.4)
Oklahoma	6,117	11.5	(10.5–12.6)	—	—	—
Oregon	4,294	7.6	(6.6–8.7)	—	—	—
Rhode Island	4,002	8.6	(7.4–9.9)	—	—	—
South Carolina	7,853	8.8	(8.0–9.7)	—	—	—
Tennessee	3,860	10.3	(9.0–11.8)	—	—	—
Texas	5,856	8.5	(7.3–9.9)	—	—	—
Utah	4,621	8.7	(7.5–10.0)	—	—	—
Vermont	6,297	7.1	(6.3–8.0)	6,185	7.8	(6.9–8.7)
Virginia	4,636	7.3	(6.0–8.9)	—	—	—
Washington	10,397	6.4	(5.8–7.1)	9,382	7.4	(6.7–8.2)
West Virginia	3,439	13.7	(12.3–15.2)	—	—	—
Wisconsin	4,228	6.7	(5.7–7.8)	—	—	—
Wyoming	4,495	7.3	(6.4–8.3)	—	—	—
Puerto Rico	4,181	11.2	(10.1–12.3)	—	—	—
U.S. Virgin Islands	2,649	7.1	(6.0–8.5)	—	—	—

Abbreviation: CI = confidence interval.

* Patient Health Questionnaire-8 depression severity score of ≥10.

† Not measured.

Table 5. Prevalence of postpartum depressive symptoms, by sociodemographic characteristics and symptoms — Pregnancy Risk Assessment Monitoring System, United States, multiple sites, 2004–2008*

	Self-reported symptoms†								
	Down, depressed, or hopeless			Little interest or pleasure in doing things			Either or both symptoms§		
Characteristic	No.	%	(95% CI)	No.	%	(95% CI)	No.	%	(95% CI)
Total	138,113	9.5	(9.2– 9.7)	137,979	9.8	(9.5–10.0)	137,461	14.5	(14.2–14.8)
Age group (yrs)									
≤19	13,266	14.3	(13.2–15.4)	13,251	15.5	(14.3–16.7)	13,209	23.3	(21.9–24.7)
20–29	70,749	10.5	(10.1–10.9)	70,699	10.6	(10.2–11.1)	70,433	15.8	(15.3–16.3)
30–39	49,724	6.7	(6.4– 7.1)	49,648	7.0	(6.6– 7.4)	49,465	10.3	(9.9–10.8)
≥40	4,365	7.5	(6.3– 8.9)	4,372	8.2	(6.9– 9.8)	4,345	12.1	(10.5–13.9)
Race/Ethnicity									
Hispanic	20,847	9.9	(9.2–10.6)	20,729	11.8	(11.0–12.6)	20,632	16.8	(15.9–17.7)
White, non-Hispanic	73,272	8.8	(8.5– 9.1)	73,362	7.5	(7.2– 7.9)	73,106	11.9	(11.6–12.3)
Black, non-Hispanic	20,307	12.1	(11.3–13.0)	20,219	15.9	(14.9–16.8)	20,184	21.5	(20.5–22.6)
Other	22,803	9.3	(8.5–10.2)	22,783	14.5	(13.5–15.6)	22,659	19.7	(18.5–20.9)

Abbreviation: CI = confidence interval.

* New York state excludes New York City, which conducts a separate survey. 2004: Alaska, Colorado, Georgia, Hawaii, Maine, Maryland, Minnesota, Nebraska, New Mexico, New York, North Carolina, Oregon, Rhode Island, South Carolina, Utah, Vermont, and Washington; 2005: Alaska, Colorado, Georgia, Hawaii, Maine, Maryland, Minnesota, Nebraska, New Mexico, New York, North Carolina, Ohio, Oregon, Rhode Island, South Carolina, Utah, Vermont, and Washington; 2006: Alaska, Colorado, Georgia, Hawaii, Maine, Maryland, Minnesota, Nebraska, New York, Ohio, Oregon, Rhode Island, South Carolina, Utah, Vermont, and Washington; 2007: Alaska, Colorado, Delaware, Georgia, Hawaii, Maine, Maryland, Massachusetts, Minnesota, Missouri, Nebraska, New York, North Carolina, Oregon, Pennsylvania, Rhode Island, South Carolina, South Dakota Tribal, Utah, Vermont, Washington, Wisconsin, and Wyoming; 2008: Alaska, Colorado, Delaware, Georgia, Hawaii, Maine, Maryland, Massachusetts,

Minnesota, Nebraska, New York, North Carolina, Ohio, Oregon, Pennsylvania, Rhode Island, Tennessee, Utah, Vermont, Washington, Wisconsin, and Wyoming.

† Survey questions: "Since your new baby was born, how often have you felt down, depressed, or hopeless?" and "Since your new baby was born, how often have you had little interest or little pleasure in doing things?" Possible responses are "never," "rarely," "sometimes," "often," and "always." Women who answered "often" or "always" were categorized as having symptoms of postpartum depression.

§ Women who answered "often" or "always" to either question or both questions.

Table 6. Prevalence of postpartum depressive symptoms, by state and symptoms — Pregnancy Risk Assessment Monitoring System, 22 states, 2008

	Self-reported symptoms*					
	Down, depressed, or hopeless		Little interest or pleasure in doing things		Either or both symptoms†	
State	%	(95% CI)	%	(95% CI)	%	(95% CI)
Alaska	8.0	(6.3–10.1)	9.1	(7.3–11.2)	13.2	(11.0–15.7)
Colorado	7.9	(6.5–9.6)	9.5	(7.9–11.4)	13.5	(11.6–15.6)
Delaware	8.8	(7.3–10.5)	9.0	(7.5–10.8)	14.4	(12.6–16.6)
Georgia	9.5	(7.0–12.8)	9.0	(6.6–12.2)	12.8	(9.9–16.5)
Hawaii	7.9	(6.7–9.4)	10.2	(8.8–11.7)	14.7	(13.1–16.5)
Maine	10.3	(8.4–12.6)	8.4	(6.7–10.5)	12.6	(10.5–15.1)
Maryland	8.9	(7.0–11.3)	8.6	(6.7–10.9)	13.5	(11.1–16.3)
Massachusetts	7.9	(6.3–9.9)	8.8	(7.3–10.6)	12.9	(10.9–15.1)
Minnesota	6.7	(5.4–8.3)	6.4	(5.1–7.9)	9.8	(8.3–11.6)
Nebraska	7.4	(5.9–9.1)	6.8	(5.5–8.4)	10.8	(9.1–12.8)
New York	7.5	(5.8–9.7)	9.4	(7.4–11.8)	12.7	(10.4–15.4)
North Carolina	10.0	(8.3–12.0)	9.2	(7.6–11.1)	14.2	(12.2–16.4)
Ohio	11.2	(9.2–13.6)	10.9	(9.0–13.3)	16.4	(14.0–19.1)

Table 6. (Continued)

	Self-reported symptoms*					
	Down, depressed, or hopeless		Little interest or pleasure in doing things		Either or both symptoms†	
State	%	(95% CI)	%	(95% CI)	%	(95% CI)
Oregon	9.0	(7.0–11.5)	7.4	(5.7–9.6)	12.3	(10.0–15.0)
Pennsylvania	7.3	(5.8–9.3)	8.8	(7.1–10.9)	12.0	(10.0–14.3)
Rhode Island	9.1	(7.4–11.2)	10.1	(8.3–12.2)	13.9	(11.8–16.3)
Tennessee	15.0	(11.9–18.7)	12.3	(9.5–15.7)	21.3	(17.7–25.4)
Utah	8.5	(7.2–10.0)	8.3	(7.1–9.8)	12.6	(11.0–14.3)
Vermont	8.7	(7.2–10.6)	6.9	(5.5–8.6)	11.7	(9.8–13.8)
Washington	8.9	(7.1–11.0)	9.6	(7.8–11.7)	13.8	(11.6–16.2)
Wisconsin	7.8	(6.2–9.9)	9.4	(7.5–11.6)	13.8	(11.6–16.3)
Wyoming	8.1	(6.3–10.4)	8.2	(6.3–10.6)	12.0	(9.7–14.7)
Total	*9.1*	*(8.5–9.7)*	*9.2*	*(8.7–9.8)*	*13.7*	*(13.1–14.4)*

Abbreviation: CI = confidence interval.

* Survey questions: "Since your new baby was born, how often have you felt down, depressed, or hopeless?" and "Since your new baby was born, how often have you had little interest or little pleasure in doing things?" Possible responses are "never," "rarely," "sometimes," "often," and "always." Women who answered "often" or "always" were categorized as having symptoms of postpartum depression.

† Women who answered "often" or "always" to either question or both questions

Table 7. Prevalence of serious psychological distress* among adults aged ≥18 years, by sociodemographic characteristics — National Health Interview Survey, United States, 2009

Characteristic	No.	%	(95% CI)
Total	27,858	3.2	(2.9–3.5)
Sex Male	12,322	2.8	(2.4–3.2)
Female	15,536	3.7	(3.3–4.1)
Age group (yrs) <45	12,846	3.3	(2.9–3.7)
45–64	9,503	3.7	(3.2–4.2)
≥65	5,509	2.1	(1.6–2.6)
Race/Ethnicity			
Hispanic	5,196	3.4	(2.9–4.0)
Black, non-Hispanic	4,374	3.8	(3.0–4.7)
White, non-Hispanic	16,187	3.2	(2.8–3.6)

Abbreviation: CI = confidence interval. *Kessler-6 score of ≥13.

Table 8. Prevalence of serious psychological distress* among adults aged ≥18 years, by sociodemographic characteristics — Behavioral Risk Factor Surveillance System, United States, 2007 and 2009

	2007†			2009§		
Characteristic	No.	%	(95% CI)	No.	%	(95% CI)
Total	203,096	4.0	(3.8–4.1)	87,992	3.9	(3.6–4.3)
Sex Male	75,450	3.5	(3.3–3.9)	33,434	3.5	(3.0–4.0)
Female	127,646	4.3	(4.1–4.6)	54,558	4.4	(4.0–4.8)
Age group (yrs)						
18–24	7,509	3.6	(3.0–4.3)	2,592	3.1	(2.1–4.5)

Table 8. (Continued)

Characteristic	2007†			2009§		
	No.	%	(95% CI)	No.	%	(95% CI)
25–34	21,168	4.0	(3.6–4.6)	7,329	4.0	(3.2–4.9)
35–44	32,612	4.2	(3.8–4.8)	11,930	3.8	(3.2–4.5)
45–54	42,859	4.6	(4.3–5.0)	17,925	4.9	(4.3–5.6)
≥55	97,652	3.4	(3.1–3.7)	47,668	3.7	(3.3–4.2)
Race/Ethnicity						
White, non-Hispanic	158,774	3.4	(3.2–3.5)	68,335	3.5	(3.2–3.9)
Black, non-Hispanic	14,364	6.1	(5.1–7.2)	8,410	5.4	(4.5–6.4)
Other, non-Hispanic¶	12,700	4.0	(3.3–4.7)	6,507	3.1	(2.3–4.1)
Hispanic	15,552	5.5	(4.8–6.3)	3,886	5.3	(4.2–6.7)

*Kessler-6 score of ≥13.

† Data from 35 states, District of Columbia, and Puerto Rico.

§ Data from 16 states.

¶ Asian, Native Hawaiian/Pacific Islander, American Indian/Alaska Native, other race, and multiple races.

Table 9. Prevalence of serious psychological distress* among adults aged ≥18 years, by state/area — Behavioral Risk Factor Surveillance System, United States, 2007 and 2009

State/Area	2007			2009		
	No.	%	(95% CI)	No.	%	(95% CI)
Alaska	2,329	2.4	(1.5–3.9)	—†	—	—
Arkansas	5,242	5.1	(4.4–6.0)	—	—	—
California	5,169	3.5	(2.9–4.3)	4,784	3.7	(3.0–4.4)
Colorado	5,460	3.2	(2.6–3.9)	—	—	—

	2007			2009		
State/Area	No.	%	(95% CI)	No.	%	(95% CI)
District of Columbia	3,545	2.6	(2.0–3.4)	—	—	—
Georgia	6,872	5.0	(4.2–5.9)	5,243	3.1	(2.5–3.9)
Hawaii	6,288	2.4	(1.9–3.0)	6,204	2.4	(1.9–2.9)
Illinois	5,043	3.0	(2.5–3.7)	—	—	—
Indiana	5,473	3.5	(2.9–4.1)	—	—	—
Iowa	4,891	2.3	(1.8–2.8)	—	—	—
Kansas	4,034	2.6	(2.0–3.3)	8,617	2.5	(2.1–3.0)
Kentucky	6,049	6.5	(5.6–7.4)	—	—	—
Louisiana	5,865	5.3	(4.6–6.1)	—	—	—
Maine	3,884	3.8	(3.1–4.7)	—	—	—
Massachusetts	4,394	3.1	(2.4–3.9)	4,738	3.3	(2.6–4.2)
Michigan	4,194	3.8	(3.1–4.7)	2,779	3.5	(2.6–4.6)
Minnesota	4,716	2.7	(2.1–3.4)			
Mississippi	7,173	6.6	(5.8–7.5)	10,113	7.1	(6.3–7.9)
Missouri	4,842	5.0	(4.2–6.0)	4,555	4.5	(3.6–5.7)
Montana	5,628	3.5	(2.9–4.2)			
Nebraska	5,103	2.5	(1.9–3.3)	4,933	2.6	(1.9–3.7)
Nevada	3,858	4.0	(3.2–5.1)	3,536	4.0	(3.0–5.1)
New Hampshire	5,613	3.2	(2.7–3.8)	—	—	—
New Mexico	5,972	4.1	(3.4–4.8)	—	—	—
Ohio	5,065	4.6	(3.8–5.5)	—	—	—
Oklahoma	6,793	5.3	(4.6–6.1)	—	—	—
Oregon	1,875	2.9	(2.2–3.8)	—	—	—
Rhode Island	3,976	4.7	(3.9–5.6)	—	—	—
South Carolina	9,583	5.0	(4.3–5.8)	8,843	4.4	(3.8–5.2)

Table 9. (Continued)

State/Area	2007			2009		
	No.	%	(95% CI)	No.	%	(95% CI)
Tennessee	—	—	—	2,216	9.4	(7.7–11.6)
Texas	7,673	5.2	(4.3–6.2)			
Utah	—	—	—	2,446	1.9	(1.4–2.6)
Vermont	6,592	3.3	(2.7–4.2)	6,278	3.1	(2.5–3.7)
Virginia	5,689	3.3	(2.7–4.0)	—	—	—
Washington	13,317	2.9	(2.5–3.4)	7,062	2.9	(2.4–3.5)
Wisconsin	4,538	2.7	(2.1–3.4)	—	—	—
Wyoming	5,738	3.2	(2.6–3.9)	5,645	2.6	(1.9–3.4)
Puerto Rico	3,776	6.0	(5.2–7.0)	—	—	—

Abbreviation: CI = confidence interval. * Kessler-6 score of ≥13. † Not measured.

Table 10. Mean number of mentally unhealthy days* during past 30 days among adults aged ≥18 years, by sociodemographic characteristics — Behavioral Risk Factor Surveillance System, United States, 2009†

Characteristic	No. of respondents	Mean no. of mentally unhealthy days	(95% CI)
Total	424,218	3.5	(3.4–3.6)
Sex			
Male	161,046	2.9	(2.8–3.1)
Female	263,172	4.0	(3.9–4.1)
Age group (yrs)			
18–24	13,032	3.9	(3.6–4.2)
25–34	36,755	3.8	(3.6–4.0)
35–44	59,253	3.7	(3.6–3.9)

Characteristic	No. of respondents	Mean no. of mentally unhealthy days	(95% CI)
45–54	85,446	3.9	(3.8–4.1)
≥55	226,168	2.8	(2.7–2.9)
Race/Ethnicity			
White, non-Hispanic	333,119	3.3	(3.2–3.4)
Black, non-Hispanic	33,741	4.1	(3.9–4.4)
Other, non-Hispanic§	23,549	3.6	(3.3–3.8)
Hispanic	29,361	3.8	(3.6–4.1)

Abbreviation: CI = confidence interval.

* Survey question: "Now thinking about your mental health, which includes stress, depression, and problems with emotions, for how many days during the past 30 days was your mental health not good?"

† Data from 50 states, Guam, Puerto Rico, and U.S. Virgin Islands. Only includes respondents interviewed in 2009.

§ Asian, Native Hawaiian/ Pacific Islander, American Indian/Alaska Native, other race, and multiple races.

Table 11. Mean number of mentally unhealthy days* during past 30 days among adults aged ≥18 years, by state/area — Behavioral Risk Factor Surveillance System, United States, 2009

State/Area	No. of respondents†	Mean no. of mentally unhealthy days	(95% CI)
Alabama	6,616	4.2	(3.8–4.5)
Alaska	2,363	2.5	(2.1–3.0)
Arizona	5,403	3.4	(3.0–3.9)
Arkansas	3,904	3.6	(3.2–4.0)
California	17,316	3.7	(3.5–3.9)
Colorado	11,768	3.1	(2.9–3.4)
Connecticut	6,414	3.1	(2.8–3.4)
Delaware	4,315	3.1	(2.8–3.5)
District of Columbia	3,844	2.7	(2.4–3.0)

Table 11. (Continued)

State/Area	No. of respondents†	Mean no. of mentally unhealthy days	(95% CI)
Florida	11,753	3.5	(3.2–3.8)
Georgia	5,761	2.8	(2.5–3.1)
Hawaii	6,642	2.6	(2.3–2.9)
Idaho	5,315	3.2	(2.9–3.5)
Illinois	5,819	3.5	(3.2–3.8)
Indiana	9,094	3.8	(3.5–4.1)
Iowa	5,941	2.6	(2.4–2.9)
Kansas	18,702	2.9	(2.7–3.1)
Kentucky	9,536	4.6	(4.2–5.0)
Louisiana	8,765	3.5	(3.2–3.8)
Maine	7,942	3.4	(3.2–3.7)
Maryland	8,440	3.3	(3.0–3.6)
Massachusetts	16,397	3.2	(2.9–3.4)
Michigan	9,103	3.7	(3.4–4.0)
Minnesota	5,583	2.8	(2.5–3.1)
Mississippi	10,997	4.1	(3.8–4.4)
Missouri	5,000	3.9	(3.5–4.3)
Montana	7,506	3.3	(3.0–3.6)
Nebraska	15,733	2.6	(2.4–2.9)
Nevada	3,791	4.0	(3.5–4.6)
New Hampshire	5,931	3.1	(2.8–3.4)
New Jersey	12,025	3.3	(3.0–3.6)
New Mexico	8,715	3.5	(3.2–3.8)
New York	6,786	3.5	(3.1–3.8)

State/Area	No. of respondents†	Mean no. of mentally unhealthy days	(95% CI)
North Carolina	13,068	3.8	(3.5–4.1)
North Dakota	4,698	2.4	(2.1–2.7)
Ohio	9,650	3.8	(3.5–4.1)
Oklahoma	7,724	4.3	(3.9–4.6)
Oregon	4,238	3.2	(2.8–3.6)
Pennsylvania	9,003	3.6	(3.3–3.9)
Rhode Island	6,223	3.4	(3.1–3.8)
South Carolina	9,568	3.5	(3.2–3.8)
South Dakota	6,739	2.4	(2.1–2.7)
Tennessee	5,510	3.8	(3.4–4.2)
Texas	11,381	3.6	(3.3–3.9)
Utah	9,997	3.3	(3.0–3.5)
Vermont	6,563	3.3	(3.1–3.6)
Virginia	5,078	3.4	(2.9–3.8)
Washington	20,018	3.3	(3.1–3.5)
West Virginia	4,761	4.1	(3.8–4.5)
Wisconsin	4,517	2.9	(2.5–3.2)
Wyoming	5,965	3.2	(2.8–3.5)
Guam	1,247	2.1	(1.6–2.5)
Puerto Rico	4,136	3.2	(2.8–3.5)
U.S. Virgin Islands	2,414	2.9	(2.4–3.3)

Abbreviation: CI = confidence interval.

* Survey question: “Now thinking about your mental health, which includes stress, depression, and problems with emotions, for how many days during the past 30 days was your mental health not good?”

† Only includes respondents interviewed in 2009.

Table 12. Percentage of adults aged ≥18 years who ever received a diagnosis of depression in their lifetime, by sociodemographic characteristics — Behavioral Risk Factor Surveillance System, United States, 2006 and 2008

	2006*			2008†		
Characteristic	No.	%	(95% CI)	No.	%	(95% CI)
Total	215,576	15.7	(15.4–16.1)	91,377	16.1	(15.6–16.6)
Sex Male	82,284	11.1	(10.6–11.5)	34,481	11.2	(10.6–11.9)
Female	133,292	20.2	(19.7–20.6)	56,896	20.7	(20.0–21.3)
Age group (yrs)						
18–24	9,652	14.5	(13.3–15.8)	3,081	14.8	(12.9–17.0)
25–34	25,525	14.4	(13.7–15.2)	8,584	14.4	(13.2–15.7)
35–44	36,586	16.7	(16.0–17.5)	13,444	16.7	(15.6–17.9)
45–54	44,877	19.3	(18.6–20.0)	18,937	19.9	(18.9–20.9)
≥55	97,304	14.4	(14.0–14.8)	46,637	14.9	(14.3–15.5)
Race/Ethnicity						
White, non-Hispanic	165,506	17.2	(16.8–17.6)	73,604	17.3	(16.8–17.8)
Black, non-Hispanic	17,650	11.2	(10.4–12.0)	5,280	12.3	(10.7–14.0)
Other, non-Hispanic§	13,245	15.1	(13.7–16.6)	6,783	12.2	(10.5–14.1)
Hispanic	17,044	12.6	(11.6–13.7)	4,807	12.8	(11.1–14.7)

Abbreviation: CI = confidence interval.

* Data from 38 states, District of Columbia, Puerto Rico, and U.S. Virgin Islands

† Data from 16 states.

§ Asian, Native Hawaiian/Pacific Islander, American Indian/Alaska Native, other race, and multiple races.

Table 13. Percentage of adults aged ≥18 years who ever received a diagnosis of depression in their lifetime, by state/area — Behavioral Risk Factor Surveillance System, United States, 2006 and 2008

	2006			2008		
State/Area	No.	%	(95% CI)	No.	%	(95% CI)
Alabama	3,111	17.4	(15.8–19.2)	—*	—	—
Alaska	1,998	17.4	(15.4–19.7)	—	—	—
Arizona	—	—	—	5,768	18.1	(16.1–20.4)
Arkansas	5,288	21.3	(19.9–22.7)	—	—	—
California	5,284	13.5	(12.4–14.7)	—	—	—
Colorado				5,463	17.7	(16.4–19.0)
Connecticut	4,446	14.3	(13.0–15.8)	—	—	—
Delaware	3,941	17.0	(15.2–18.9)	—	—	—
District of Columbia	3,754	15.0	(13.5–16.6)	—	—	—
Florida	10,232	13.1	(12.2–14.2)	—	—	—
Georgia	6,992	14.5	(13.4–15.6)	—	—	—
Hawaii	6,229	8.8	(8.0–9.8)	6,218	9.8	(8.9–10.8)
Idaho	—	—	—	4,893	18.9	(17.4–20.4)
Illinois	—	—	—	5,047	13.5	(12.4–14.7)
Indiana	6,208	19.8	(18.6–21.1)	—	—	—
Iowa	5,164	14.7	(13.5–15.9)	—	—	—
Kansas	4,109	14.1	(12.8–15.6)	4,125	13.5	(12.2–14.8)
Louisiana	6,725	13.2	(12.3–14.2)	5,893	12.4	(11.4–13.4)
Maine	3,864	19.9	(18.5–21.5)	3,981	20.9	(19.3–22.6)
Maryland	4,577	15.4	(13.9–17.1)			
Massachusetts	—	—	—	6,326	15.3	(14.0–16.7)
Michigan	5,484	15.9	(14.7–17.0)	—	—	—

Table 13. (Continued)

State/Area	2006			2008		
	No.	%	(95% CI)	No.	%	(95% CI)
Minnesota	4,232	14.4	(13.2–15.8)	—	—	—
Mississippi	5,828	16.9	(15.7–18.2)	6,990	16.8	(15.7–18.1)
Missouri	5,045	18.4	(16.8–20.1)	—	—	—
Montana	5,733	17.1	(15.9–18.4)	—	—	—
Nebraska	3,851	15.5	(13.8–17.3)	5,221	16.9	(15.0–19.1)
Nevada	3,442	15.5	(13.9–17.3)	—	—	—
New Hampshire	5,592	17.2	(16.0–18.6)	—	—	—
New Mexico	6,146	17.1	(16.0–18.3)	—	—	—
New York	—	—	—	3,692	15.5	(14.2–16.9)
North Carolina	—	—	—			
North Dakota	4,566	16.8	(15.4–18.4)	4,865	15.0	(13.6–16.4)
Ohio				6,230	19.5	(18.1–20.9)
Oklahoma	6,786	19.9	(18.7–21.1)	—	—	—
Oregon	4,670	21.3	(19.9–22.7)	—	—	—
Rhode Island	4,267	16.8	(15.3–18.4)	—	—	—
South Carolina	8,703	17.3	(16.3–18.4)	—	—	—
Tennessee	4,172	16.4	(14.8–18.0)	—	—	—
Texas	6,395	15.4	(13.9–17.0)	—	—	—
Utah	4,983	19.6	(18.1–21.2)	—	—	—
Vermont	6,794	20.2	(19.1–21.4)	6,586	21.4	(20.2–22.7)
Virginia	5,133	15.1	(13.7–16.7)	—	—	—
Washington	11,301	20.1	(19.1–21.1)	10,079	17.2	(16.2–18.1)
West Virginia	3,725	20.2	(18.7–21.7)	—	—	—

State/Area	2006			2008		
	No.	%	(95% CI)	No.	%	(95% CI)
Wisconsin	4,375	16.4	(15.0–17.8)	—	—	—
Wyoming	4,818	18.2	(17.0–19.5)	—	—	—
Puerto Rico	4,588	18.1	(16.9–19.5)	—	—	—
U.S. Virgin Islands	3,025	6.8	(5.8–7.9)	—	—	—

Abbreviation:

CI = confidence interval.

* Not measured.

Table 14. Percentage of adults aged ≥18 years who ever received a diagnosis of anxiety in their lifetime, by sociodemographic characteristics — Behavioral Risk Factor Surveillance System, United States, 2006 and 2008

Characteristic	2006*			2008†		
	No.	%	(95% CI)	No.	%	(95% CI)
Total	215,522	11.3	(11.0–11.6)	91,339	12.3	(11.8–12.7)
Sex Male	82,288	8.2	(7.8–8.7)	34,447	9.1	(8.5–9.7)
Female	133,234	14.3	(13.9–14.6)	56,892	15.2	(14.6–15.9)
Age group (yrs)						
18–24	9,660	11.3	(10.2–12.5)	3,079	13.0	(11.2–15.1)
25–34	25,530	11.6	(10.9–12.3)	8,574	11.9	(10.8–13.1)
35–44	36,589	12.0	(11.4–12.7)	13,443	13.6	(12.5–14.7)
45–54	44,868	12.9	(12.3–13.5)	18,945	14.1	(13.2–15.0)
≥55	97,246	9.8	(9.5–10.2)	46,606	10.3	(9.8–10.8)
Race/Ethnicity						
White, non-Hispanic	165,498	12.2	(11.9–12.5)	73,577	12.9	(12.5–13.4)
Black, non-Hispanic	17,634	8.6	(7.8–9.4)	5,270	9.3	(7.9–10.8)

Table 14. (Continued)

Characteristic	2006* No.	2006* %	2006* (95% CI)	2008† No.	2008† %	2008† (95% CI)
Other, non-Hispanic§	13,231	12.0	(10.6–13.7)	6,781	11.8	(9.9–13.9)
Hispanic	17,041	9.0	(8.2–9.8)	4,806	9.7	(8.2–11.3)

Abbreviation: CI = confidence interval.

* Data from 38 states, District of Columbia, Puerto Rico, and U.S. Virgin Islands.

† Data from 16 states.

§ Asian, Native Hawaiian/Pacific Islander, American Indian/Alaska Native, other race, and multiple races.

Table 15. Percentage of adults aged ≥18 years who ever received a diagnosis of anxiety in their lifetime, by state/area — Behavioral Risk Factor Surveillance System, United States, 2006 and 2008

State/Area	2006 No.	2006 %	2006 (95% CI)	2008 No.	2008 %	2008 (95% CI)
Alabama	3,107	14.0	(12.5–15.7)	—*	—	—
Alaska	2,000	12.0	(10.2–14.1)	—	—	—
Arizona		14.0	(12.8–15.2)	5,777	13.0	(11.2–15.1)
Arkansas	5,285			—	—	—
California	5,283	9.6	(8.6–10.7)	—	—	—
Colorado				5,462	12.3	(11.1–13.5)
Connecticut	4,451	10.0	(8.9–11.3)	—	—	—
Delaware	3,935	12.1	(10.5–13.9)	—	—	—
District of Columbia	3,758	9.5	(8.3–10.9)	—	—	—
Florida	10,241	11.2	(10.3–12.2)	—	—	—
Georgia	6,997	11.1	(10.1–12.1)	—	—	—

	2006			2008		
State/Area	No.	%	(95% CI)	No.	%	(95% CI)
Hawaii	6,222	8.0	(7.2–8.9)	6,212	8.3	(7.4–9.2)
Idaho	—	—	—	4,896	11.6	(10.4–12.9)
Illinois	—	—	—	5,044	10.8	(9.7–12.0)
Indiana	6,209	13.8	(12.7–15.0)	—	—	—
Iowa	5,173	9.1	(8.2–10.1)	—	—	—
Kansas	4,110	9.9	(8.8–11.2)	4,128	10.4	(9.2–11.7)
Louisiana	6,719	10.9	(10.0–11.8)	5,896	11.5	(10.5–12.6)
Maine	3,863	16.1	(14.5–17.7)	3,986	16.7	(15.2–18.4)
Maryland	4,582	10.9	(9.6–12.4)			
Massachusetts	—	—	—	6,289	13.9	(12.6–15.2)
Michigan	5,487	11.1	(10.1–12.1)	—	—	—
Minnesota	4,232	10.1	(9.1–11.3)	—	—	—
Mississippi	5,808	13.7	(12.6–14.8)	6,984	13.1	(12.1–14.3)
Missouri	5,044	12.5	(11.0–14.3)	—	—	—
Montana	5,735	10.9	(9.8–12.0)	—	—	—
Nebraska	3,850	9.8	(8.4–11.4)	5,223	10.6	(8.9–12.5)
Nevada	3,434	11.6	(10.2–13.2)	—	—	—
New Hampshire	5,604	12.8	(11.7–14.0)	—	—	—
New Jersey	—	—	—	—	—	—
New Mexico	6,155	12.0	(11.0–13.1)	—	—	—
New York	—	—	—	3,692	12.2	(11.0–13.5)
North Dakota	4,564	10.2	(9.0–11.6)	4,868	10.7	(9.4–12.1)
Ohio	—	—	—	6,226	13.8	(12.6–15.2)
Oklahoma	6,775	14.8	(13.8–15.9)	—	—	—
Oregon	4,667	13.2	(12.1–14.5)	—	—	—

Table 15. (Continued)

State/Area	2006			2008		
	No.	%	(95% CI)	No.	%	(95% CI)
Rhode Island	4,266	13.2	(12.0–14.6)	—	—	—
South Carolina	8,694	12.9	(12.0–13.8)	—	—	—
Tennessee	4,171	12.2	(10.7–13.8)	—	—	—
Texas	6,386	10.3	(9.1–11.8)	—	—	—
Utah	4,982	12.6	(11.4–14.0)	—	—	—
Vermont	6,782	14.2	(13.2–15.2)	6,579	14.6	(13.6–15.7)
Virginia	5,135	10.7	(9.5–12.1)	—	—	—
Washington	11,285	12.9	(12.0–13.8)	10,077	11.8	(11.0–12.7)
West Virginia	3,717	17.2	(15.8–18.7)	—	—	—
Wisconsin	4,377	10.2	(9.1–11.5)	—	—	—
Wyoming	4,815	10.6	(9.6–11.7)	—	—	—
Puerto Rico	4,594	14.8	(13.6–16.0)	—	—	—
U.S. Virgin Islands	3,028	5.4	(4.6–6.4)	—	—	—

Abbreviation: CI = confidence interval. * Not measured.

Table 16. Percentage of adults aged ≥18 years who ever received a diagnosis of bipolar disorder or schizophrenia,* by sociodemographic characteristics — National Health Interview Survey, United States, 2007

	Frequency	Bipolar disorder		Schizophrenia	
		%	(SE)	%	(SE)
Total	23,354	1.7	(0.1)	0.6	(0.1)
Sex Male	10,356	1.4	(0.1)	0.8	(0.2)
Female	12,998	1.9	(0.2)	0.4	(0.1)

	Frequency	Bipolar disorder		Schizophrenia	
		%	(SE)	%	(SE)
Age group (yrs)					
18–39	8,852	2.2	(0.2)	0.6	(0.2)
40–54	6,529	1.9	(0.2)	0.7	(0.1)
≥55	7,973	0.8	(0.1)	0.5	(0.1)
Race/Ethnicity Hispanic	4,191	0.9	(0.2)	0.5	(0.1)
White, non-Hispanic	14,030	1.9	(0.1)	0.6	(0.1)
Black, non-Hispanic	3,697	1.3	(0.2)	0.8	(0.2)

Abbreviation: SE = standard error.

*Bipolar disorder and schizophrenia are not mutually exclusive.

Table 17. Annual average number and rate of ambulatory care visits* for mental health disorders among adults aged ≥18 years, by diagnosis and medical setting — National Ambulatory Medical Care Survey (NAMCS) and National Hospital Ambulatory Medical Care Survey (NHAMCS), United States, 2007–2008

						Medical setting					
						Physician office (NAMCS)		OPD (NHAMCS)		ED (NHAMCS)	
Primary diagnosis group†	ICD-9-CM codes	No. visits (in thousands)	(SE) (in thousands)	Rate of visits§	(SE)	%	(SE)	%	(SE)	%	(SE)
All diagnoses		961,646	(28,861)	42,982	(1,290)	82.3	(0.9)	8.0	(0.7)	9.7	(0.4)
Mental health disorders	290–319	47,835	(2,534)	2,138	(113)	80.7	(1.6)	11.8	(1.5)	7.5	(0.5)
Schizophrenic disorders	295	2,730	(507)	122		79.4	(4.5)	13.4	(3.3)	7.2	(1.6)
Major depressive disorder	296.2–296.3	7,530	(793)	337	(35)	85.0	(2.7)	13.6	(2.6)	1.4	(0.3)
Other psychoses	290–294, 296.0–296.1, 296.4–299	8,451	(584)	378	(26)	80.8	(2.0)	11.0	(1. 8)	8.3	(0.8)
Anxiety states	300.0	6,679	(544)	299		84.7	(1.5)	7.0	(1.1)	8.3	(0.9)

Table 17. (Continued)

						Medical setting					
						Physician office (NAMCS)		OPD (NHAMCS)		ED (NHAMCS)	
Primary diagnosis group†	ICD-9-CM codes	No. visits (in thousands)	(SE) (in thousands)	Rate of visits§	(SE)	%	(SE)	%	(SE)	%	(SE)
Neurotic depression	300.4	3,231	(323)	144	(14)	89.6	(1.7)	8.4	(1.6)	2.0	(0.5)
Alcohol dependence syndrome	303	653	(116)	29	(5)	—¶	(7.4)	38.7	(7.2)	23.5	(4.8)
Drug dependence and nondependent use of drugs	304–305	3,164	(459)	141		40.3	(6.5)	29.8	(7.4)	29.9	(4.5)
Acute reaction to stress and adjustment reaction	308–309	2,778	(308)	124	(14)	81.8	(3.2)	14.5	(3.1)	3.7	(0.7)
Depressive disorder, not elsewhere classified	311	7,299	(622)	326	(28)	85.8	(1.7)	7.9	(1.3)	6.4	(0.8)
Attention deficit disorder	314.0	1,736	(242)	78	(11)	94.6	(1.4)	5.4	(1.4)	—	(0.0)
Other mental disorders	300.1–300.3, 300.5–300.9, 301–302, 306–307, 310, 312–313, 314.1–319	3,585	(494)	160		83.1	(2.7)	8.5	(1.7)	8.4	(1.5)

Abbreviations: ED = emergency department; ICD-9-CM = International Classification of Diseases, Ninth Revision, Clinical Modification; OPD = outpatient department;

SE = standard error.

* Visits to physician offices and hospital outpatient and emergency departments.

† Primary diagnosis groups are based on a reclassification of codes.

§ Rate per 10,000 persons, based on U.S. Census Bureau estimates of the civilian noninstitutionalized adult population as of July 1, 2007, and July 1, 2008. Additional information on calculation of rates available at http://www.cdc.gov/nchs/ahcd.htm.

¶ Number does not meet standards of reliability or precision.

Table 18. Annual average number and rate of ambulatory care visits* for mental health disorders† among adults aged ≥18 years, by age group, sex, and medical setting — National Ambulatory Medical Care Survey (NAMCS) and National Hospital Ambulatory Medical Care Survey (NHAMCS), United States, 2007–2008

	No. (in thousands) and % of visits												Rate§ of visits							
	All three settings			Physician office (NAMCS)			OPD (NHAMCS)			ED (NHAMCS)			All three settings		Physician office (NAMCS)		OPD (NHAMCS)		ED (NHAMCS)	
Characteristic	No.	(SE)	%	No.	(SE)	%	No.	(SE)	%	No.	(SE)	%	Rate	(SE)	Rate	(SE)	Rate	(SE)	Rate	(SE)
Total	47,835	(—)	100	38,621	(—)	80.7	5,630	(—)	11.8	3,584	(—)	7.5	2,138	(—)	1,726	(—)	252	(—)	160	(—)
Age group (yrs)																				
18–44	22,443	(1,203)	100	17,303	(1,104)	77.1	3,070	(443)	13.7	2,070	(118)	9.2	2,036	(109)	1,570	(100)	279	(40)	188	(11)
45–64	19,451	(1,291)	100	16,205	(1,268)	83.3	2,086	(260)	10.7	1,160	(74)	6.0	2,533	(168)	2,110	(165)	272	(34)	151	
≥65	5,941	(493)	100	5,113	(489)	86.1	474	(76)	8.0	354	(40)	6.0	1,617	(134)	1,392	(133)	129	(21)	96	
Sex																				
Male	18,463	(1,206)	100	14,422	(1,170)	78.1	2,194	(308)	11.9	1,847	(105)	10.0	1,710	(112)	1,336	(108)	203	(29)	171	(10)
Female	29,372	(1,584)	100	24,199	(1,511)	82.4	3,436	(425)	11.7	1,737	(105)	5.9	2,537	(137)	2,090	(131)	297	(37)	150	(9)

Abbreviations: ED = emergency department; ICD-9-CM = International Classification of Diseases, Ninth Revision, Clinical Modification; OPD = outpatient department; SE = standard error. * Visits to physician offices and hospital outpatient and emergency departments.

† Visits with a primary diagnosis of a mental health disorder (ICD-9-CM codes 290–319).

§ Rate per 10,000 persons, based on U.S. Census Bureau estimates of the civilian noninstitutionalized population as of July 1, 2007, and July 1, 2008.

Table 19. Hospital* discharge rates† among adults aged ≥18 years with mental illness as primary discharge diagnosis, by age group, diagnosis, and sex — National Hospital Discharge Survey, United States, 2007

Primary discharge diagnosis	Age group (yrs)																	
	18–44						45–64						≥65					
	Men		Women		Total		Men		Women		Total		Men		Women		Total	
	Rate	(SE)	Rate	(SE)	Rate	(SE)	Rate	(SE)	Rate	(SE)	Rate	(SE)	Rate	(SE)	Rate	(SE)	Rate	(SE)
Adult mental illness§	105.7	(14.4)	90.1	(14.7)	97.9	(14.2)	104.9	(12.0)	88.9	(11.4)	96.7	(11.1)	63.7	(9.2)	64.9	(7.0)	64.4	(7.2)
Alcohol and drug use disorders¶	32.4	(5.0)	17.5	(3.1)	25.0	(4.0)	44.6	(5.5)	15.4	(2.1)	29.7	(3.6)	12.9	(1.8)	7.6	(1.4)	9.8	(1.2)
Schizophrenia**	18.2	(2.4)	10.4	(1.7)	14.3	(1.9)	17.0	(2.4)	17.1	(3.1)	17.1	(2.3)	5.4	(1.4)	6.6	(1.2)	6.1	(1.0)
Mood disorders††	41.5	(6.8)	50.6	(9.7)	46.0	(8.0)	32.8	(4.7)	44.4	(7.2)	38.7	(5.8)	14.7	(2.4)	22.5	(3.4)	19.2	(2.6)
Anxiety, stress, and adjustment disorders§§	3.8	(0.7)	4.5	(0.6)	4.1	(0.5)	2.6	(0.5)	4.7	(0.9)	3.7	(0.5)	1.2	(0.3)	5.3	(1.0)	3.6	(0.6)

Abbreviations: ICD-9-CM = International Classification of Diseases, Ninth Revision, Clinical Modification; SE = standard error.

* Nonfederal, short-stay (<30 days) hospitals.

† Per 10,000 persons, based on U.S. Census Bureau estimates of the civilian noninstitutionalized adult population as of July 1, 2007.

§ ICD-9-CM codes 290–312.

¶ ICD-9-CM codes 291, 292, 303, 304, and 305 (excluding 305.1).

** ICD-9-CM code 295.

†† ICD-9-CM codes 296, 300.4, and 311.

§§ ICD-9-CM codes 300.0, 300.2, 300.3, 308, and 309.

Table 20. Hospital* discharge rates† among adults aged ≥18 years with mental illness among any discharge diagnoses, by age group, diagnosis, and sex — National Hospital Discharge Survey, United States, 2007

Age group (yrs)

Discharge diagnosis (among any listed diagnoses)	18–44						45–64						≥65					
	Men		Women		Total		Men		Women		Total		Men		Women		Total	
	Rate	(SE)	Rate	(SE)	Rate	(SE)	Rate	(SE)	Rate	(SE)	Rate	(SE)	Rate	(SE)	Rate	(SE)	Rate	(SE)
Adult mental illness§	220.3	(16.7)	242.7	(18.3)	231.4	(17.0)	394.1	(22.5)	349.2	(20.2)	371.1	(20.4)	580.1	(42.3)	702.3	(38.0)	650.8	(37.6)
Alcohol and drug use disorders¶	107.2	(9.8)	74.7	(7.7)	91.1	(8.6)	166.9	(11.7)	70.9	(5.7)	117.7	(8.2)	90.4	(5.4)	40.7	(3.4)	61.6	(3.5)
Schizophrenia**	24.3	(2.6)	16.1	(1.9)	20.2	(2.1)	32.9	(3.2)	30.1	(3.4)	31.5	(2.8)	19.7	(2.7)	22.2	(2.4)	21.1	(2.1)
Mood disorders††	78.3	(9.8)	125.5	(13.1)	101.7	(11.1)	110.1	(9.8)	163.1	(11.4)	137.3	(10.0)	114.0	(9.5)	219.2	(14.6)	174.9	(11.4)
Anxiety, stress, and adjustment disorders§§	23.2	(2.7)	42.1	(4.1)	32.5	(3.1)	32.6	(2.5)	52.9	(4.1)	43.0	(3.1)	48.5	(3.8)	84.5	(5.5)	69.3	(4.1)

Abbreviations: ICD-9-CM = International Classification of Diseases, Ninth Revision, Clinical Modification; SE = standard error.

* Nonfederal, short-stay (<30 days) hospitals.

† Per 10,000 persons, based on U.S. Census Bureau estimates of the civilian noninstitutionalized adult population as of July 1, 2007.

§ ICD-9-CM codes 290–312.

¶ ICD-9-CM codes 291, 292, 303, 304, and 305 (excluding 305.1).

** ICD-9-CM code 295.

†† ICD-9-CM codes 296, 300.4, and 311.

§§ ICD-9-CM codes 300.0, 300.2, 300.3, 308, and 309.

Table 21. Percentage of nursing home residents aged ≥65 years with primary diagnosis of mental illness, by age group, diagnosis, and sex — National Nursing Home Survey, United States, 2004

	Age group (yrs)																	
	65–74						75–84						≥85					
	Men		Women		Total		Men		Women		Total		Men		Women		Total	
Primary diagnosis	%	(SE)	%	(SE)	%	(SE)	%	(SE)	%	(SE)	%	(SE)	%	(SE)	%	(SE)	%	(SE)
Alzheimer disease*	4.3	(1.0)	8.2	(1.1)	6.5	(0.8)	11.8	(1.2)	13.7	(0.8)	13.2	(0.7)	9.5	(1.1)	12.6	(0.6)	12.0	(0.6)
All adult mental illness†	16.9	(1.8)	20.0	(1.7)	18.7	(1.3)	18.8	(1.4)	20.4	(0.9)	20.0	(0.8)	21.3	(1.5)	23.9	(0.8)	23.5	(0.7)
Dementia§	7.5	(1.2)	7.0	(1.0)	7.2	(0.8)	13.2	(1.1)	13.9	(0.8)	13.7	(0.7)	15.6	(1.3)	19.2	(0.8)	18.6	(0.7)
Alcohol and drug use disorders¶	0.8	(0.4)	0.3	(0.2)	0.5	(0.2)	0.6	(0.3)	0.1	(0.1)	0.2	(0.1)	—¶¶	—¶¶	—	—	—	—
Schizophrenia**	3.4	(0.8)	5.9	(1.0)	4.8	(0.7)	1.5	(0.4)	2.2	(0.3)	2.0	(0.3)	—	—	0.5	(0.1)	0.5	(0.1)
Mood disorders††	1.6	(0.6)	3.2	(0.7)	2.5	(0.4)	1.4	(0.4)	2.2	(0.3)	1.9	(0.2)	2.1	(0.5)	1.8	(0.2)	1.9	(0.2)
Anxiety, stress, and adjustment disorders§§	0.3	(0.2)	1.3	(0.4)	0.9	(0.3)	0.1	(0.1)	0.5	(0.1)	0.4	(0.1)	0.5	(0.3)	0.3	(0.1)	0.3	(0.1)

Abbreviations: ICD-9-CM = International Classification of Diseases, Ninth Revision, Clinical Modification; SE = standard error.

* ICD-9-CM code 331.0.

† ICD-9-CM codes 290–312.

§ ICD-9-CM codes 290 and 294.

¶ ICD-9-CM codes 291, 292, 303, 304, and 305 (excluding 305.1).

** ICD-9-CM code 295.

††ICD-9-CM codes 296, 300.4, and 311.

§§ICD-9-CM codes 300.0, 300.2, 300.3, 308, and 309.

¶¶ Estimate is unreliable. Relative standard error >30%.

Table 22. Percentage of nursing home residents aged ≥65 years with any diagnosis of mental illness among all diagnoses, by age group, diagnosis, and sex — National Nursing Home Survey, United States, 2004

	Age group (yrs)																	
	65–74						75–84						≥85					
Mental health diagnosis	Men		Women		Total		Men		Women		Total		Men		Women		Total	
(among all diagnoses)	%	(SE)	%	(SE)	%	(SE)	%	(SE)	%	(SE)	%	(SE)	%	(SE)	%	(SE)	%	(SE)
Alzheimer disease*	6.8	(1.1)	12.3	(1.3)	10.0	(0.9)	17.0	(1.3)	19.2	(0.9)	18.5	(0.8)	15.7	(1.3)	18.9	(0.7)	18.4	(0.7)
All adult mental illness†	60.4	(2.4)	62.5	(2.0)	61.6	(1.6)	62.7	(1.6)	67.4	(1.1)	66.0	(1.0)	63.2	(1.8)	68.7	(0.9)	67.7	(0.8)
Dementia§	25.1	(2.0)	24.5	(1.7)	24.8	(1.3)	35.9	(1.6)	34.5	(1.1)	34.9	(0.9)	38.3	(1.7)	41.6	(0.9)	41.0	(0.9)
Alcohol and drug use disorders¶	5.6	(1.1)	1.9	(0.5)	3.5	(0.6)	2.2	(0.5)	0.7	(0.2)	1.2	(0.2)	—¶¶	—	—	—	0.5	(0.1)
Schizophrenia**	7.3	(1.2)	12.0	(1.4)	10.0	(1.0)	4.2	(0.7)	4.6	(0.5)	4.5	(0.4)	—	—	1.2	(0.2)	1.1	(0.2)
Mood disorders††	33.3	(2.3)	34.6	(1.9)	34.0	(1.5)	30.0	(1.5)	39.4	(1.1)	36.6	(1.0)	31.0	(1.6)	36.2	(0.9)	35.3	(0.8)
Anxiety, stress, and adjustment disorders§§	10.0	(1.3)	12.9	(1.3)	11.7	(0.9)	7.2	(0.8)	14.4	(0.8)	12.2	(0.6)	8.1	(1.0)	12.5	(0.6)	11.7	(0.5)

Abbreviations: ICD-9-CM = International Classification of Diseases, Ninth Revision, Clinical Modification; SE = standard error.

* ICD-9-CM code 331.0.

† ICD-9-CM codes 290–312.

§ ICD-9-CM codes 290 and 294.

¶ ICD-9-CM codes 291, 292, 303, 304, and 305 (excluding 305.1).

** ICD-9-CM code 295.

††ICD-9-CM codes 296, 300.4, and 311.

§§ICD-9-CM codes 300.0, 300.2, 300.3, 308, and 309.

¶¶ Estimate is unreliable. Relative standard error >30%.

ACKNOWLEDGMENT

This report is based, in part, on contributions by Shilpa Bengeri, Nova Research Company, Hyattsville, Maryland; Janet R. Cummings, PhD, Emory University Rollins School of Public Health, Atlanta, Georgia; Joseph Gfroerer, Center for Behavioral Health Statistics and Quality, Substance Abuse and Mental Health Services Administration, Rockville, Maryland; Elsie Freeman, MD, Maine Department of Health and Human Services, Augusta, Maine; Catherine Simile, PhD, Patricia Barnes, MA, Vladislav Beresovsky, PhD, Yelena Gorina, MPH, MS, Xiang Liu, MS, Susan M. Schappert, MA, Betzaida Tejada-Vera, Anita Bercovitz, PhD, and Jennifer H. Madans, PhD, National Center for Health Statistics, Rosemarie Kobau, MPH, MAPP, Matthew M. Zack, MD, Sherry Farr, PhD, John P. Barile, and Janet B. Croft, PhD, National Center for Chronic Disease Prevention and Health Promotion, Ruth Perou, PhD, National Center for Birth Defects and Developmental Disabilities, James W. Buehler, MD, and JM (Sally) Lin, PhD, Public Health Surveillance Program Office, Hao Tian, PhD, National Center for Emerging and Zoonotic Infectious Diseases, Ileana Arias, PhD, Office of the Director, and Stephen B. Thacker, MD, Office of Surveillance, Epidemiology, and Laboratory Services, CDC.

REFERENCES

[1] US Department of Health and Human Services. Mental health: a report of the Surgeon General. Rockville, MD: US Department of Health and Human Services, Substance Abuse and Mental Health Services Administration, Center for Mental Health Services, National Institutes of Health, National Institute of Mental Health; 1999. Available at http://www.surgeongeneral.gov/library/mentalhealth/home.html.Accessed July 1, 2011.

[2] World Health Organization. Promoting mental health: concepts, emerging evidence, practice (summary report). Geneva, Switzerland: World Health Organization; 2004. Available at http://www.who.int/mental_health/evidence/en/promoting_mhh.pdf. Accessed July 1, 2011.

[3] Kessler RC, Berglund P, Demler O, Jin R, Merikangas KR, Walters EE. Lifetime prevalence and age-of-onset distributions of DSM-IV disorders

in the National Comorbidity Survey Replication. *Arch. Gen. Psych.* 2005;62:593–602.

[4] Kessler RC, Chiu WT, Demler O, Walter EE. Prevalence, severity, and comorbidity of 12-month DSM-IV disorders in the National Comorbidity Survey Replication. *Arch. Gen. Psych.* 2005;62:617–709.

[5] Kessler RC, Chiu WT, Colpe L, et al. The prevalence and correlates of serious mental illness (SMI) in the National Comorbidity Survey Replication (NCS-R) [Chapter 15]. In Manderscheid RW, Berry JT, eds. Mental health, United States, 2004. Rockville, MD: Substance Abuse and Mental Health Services Administration; 2006. DHHS Pub no. (SMA)-06-4195.

[6] Colton CW, Manderscheid RW. Congruencies in increased mortality rates, years of potential life lost, and causes of death among public mental health clients in eight states. *Prev. Chron. Dis.* 2006;3:A42.

[7] Mathers CD, Loncar, D. Projections of global mortality and burden of disease from 2002 to 2030. *PLoS Medicine* 2006;3:e442.

[8] Murray CJ, Lopez A D. Global mortality, disability, and the contribution of risk factors: Global Burden of Disease Study. *Lancet* 1997; 349:1436–42.

[9] Kessler RC, Berglund PA, Zhao S, et al. The 12-month prevalence and correlates of serious mental illness, In Manderscheid RW, Sonnenschein MA, eds. Mental health, United States, 1996. Washington, DC: US Government Printing Office; 1996. DHHS publication no. (SMA) 96-3098.

[10] Insel TR. Assessing the economic costs of serious mental illness. *Am. J. Psych.* 2008;165:663–5.

[11] Mark TL, Levit KR, Buck JA, Coffey RM, Vandivort-Warren R. Mental health treatment expenditure trends, 1986–2003. *Psychiatr. Serv.* 2007;58:1041–8.

[12] Kessler RC, Heeringa S, Lakoma MD, Petukhova M, Rupp AE, Schoenbaum M. Individual and societal effects of mental disorders on earnings in the United States: results from the National Comorbidity Survey Replication. *Am. J. Psychiatry* 2008;165:703–11.

[13] Chapman DP, Perry GS, Strine TW. The vital link between chronic disease and depressive disorders. *Prev. Chronic. Dis.* 2005;2:A14.

[14] Evans DL, Charney DS, Lewis L, Golden RN, Gorman JM, Krishnan KR. Mood disorders in the medically ill: scientific review and recommendations. *Biol. Psychiatry* 2005;58:175–89.

[15] El-Gabalawy R, Katz LY, Sareen J. Comorbidity and associated severity of borderline personality disorder and physical health conditions in a nationally representative sample. *Psychosom. Med.* 2010;72:641–7.

[16] Lichtman JH, Bigger JT, Blumenthal JA, Frasure-Smith N, Kaufmann PG, Lespérance F. Depression and coronary heart disease: recommendations for screening, referral, and treatment: a science advisory from the American Heart Association Prevention Committee of the Council on Cardiovascular Nursing, Council on Clinical Cardiology, Council on Epidemiology and Prevention, and Interdisciplinary Council on Quality of Care and Outcomes Research: endorsed by the American Psychiatric Association. *Circulation* 2008;118:1768–75.

[17] Pincus H, Watkins K, Houtsinger J, Keyser D. Applying the Institute of Medicine quality chasm framework to improving health care for mental and substance use conditions. *Psychiatr. Clin. North Am.* 2008;31:43–56.

[18] Broadbent E, Kydd R., Sanders D, Vanderpyl J. Unmet needs and treatment seeking in high users of mental health services: role of illness perceptions. *Aust. NZJ Psychiatry* 2008;42:147–53.

[19] Levinson D, Karger CJ, Haklai Z. Chronic physical conditions and use of health services among persons with mental disorders: results from the Israel National Health Survey. *Gen. Hosp. Psychiatry* 2008;30:226–32.

[20] Shen C, Sambamoorthi U, Rust G. Co-occurring mental illness and health care utilization and expenditures in adults with obesity and chronic physical illness. *Disease Management* 2008;11:153–60.

[21] Wan JJ, Morabito DJ, Khaw J, Knudson MM, Dicker RA. Mental illness as an independent risk factor for unintentional injury and injury recidivism. *J. Trauma* 2006;61:1299–304.

[22] Hiroeh U, Appleby L, Mortensen PB, Dunn G. Death by homicide, suicide and other unnatural causes in people with mental illness: a population-based study. *Lancet* 2001;358:2110–2.

[23] Lasser K, Boyd JW, Woolhandler S, Himmelstein DU, McCormick D, Dor DH. Smoking and mental illness: a population-based prevalence study. *JAMA* 2000;284:2606–10.

[24] CDC. Updated guidelines for evaluating public health surveillance systems: recommendations from the guidelines working group. *MMWR* 2001;50(No. RR-13).

[25] Teutsch SM, Churchill RE. Principles and practice of public health surveillance. 2nd ed. New York, NY: Oxford University Press; 2000.

[26] CDC. Framework for evaluating public health surveillance systems for early detection of outbreaks. Recommendations from the CDC working group. *MMWR* 2004;53(No. RR-5).

[27] Norris FH, Galea S, Friedman MJH, Watson PJ, eds. Methods for disaster mental health research. New York, NY: Guilford Press; 2006.

[28] American Psychiatric Association. Diagnostic and statistical manual for mental disorders. 4th ed. Washington, DC: American Psychiatric Association; 2000.

[29] World Health Organization. The ICD-10 classification of mental and behavioural disorders. Clinical descriptions and diagnostic guidelines. Geneva, Switzerland: World Health Organization; 1992. Available at http://www.who.int/substance_abuse/terminology/ICD10ClinicalDiagnosis.pdf. Accessed June 4, 2011.

[30] Miller G, Holden C. Proposed revisions to psychiatry's canon unveiled. *Science* 2010;327:770–1.

[31] First MB, Spitzer RL, Gibbon M, Williams JBW. Structured Clinical Interview for DSM-IV-TR axis I disorders, Research version. New York, NY: Biometrics Research, New York State Psychiatric Institute; 2002.

[32] Kessler RC, Ustun TB. The World Mental Health (WMH) Survey Initiative Version of the World Health Organization (WHO) Composite International Diagnostic Interview (CIDI). *Int. J. Methods Psychiatr. Res.* 2004;13:93–121.

[33] Lowe B, Spitzer RL, Grafe K, et al. Comparative validity of three screening questionnaires for DSM-IV depressive disorders and physicians' diagnoses. *J. Affect. Disord.* 2004;78:131–40.

[34] Patel V, Araya R, Chowdhary N, et al. Detecting common mental disorders in primary care in India: a comparison of five screening questionnaires. *Psychol. Med.* 2008;38:221–8.

[35] O'Connor WD, Parslow RA. Mental health scales and psychiatric diagnoses: Responses to GHQ-12, K-10 and CIDI across the lifespan. *J. Affect. Disord.* 2010;121:263–7.

[36] Kroenke K, Strine TW, Spitzer RL, Williams JB, Berry JT, Mokdad AH. The PHQ-8 as a measure of current depression in the general population. *J. Affect. Disord.* 2009;114:163–73.

[37] Kroenke K, Spitzer RL, Williams JB. The PHQ-9: validity of a brief depression severity measure. *J. Gen. Intern. Med.* 2001;16:606–13.

[38] Diez-Quevedo C, Rangil T, Sanchez-Planell L, Kroenke K, Spitzer RL. Validation and utility of the Patient Health Questionnaire in diagnosing

mental disorders in 1003 general hospital Spanish inpatients. *Psychosom. Med.* 2001;63:679–86.

[39] Huang FY, Chung H, Kroenke K, Delucchi KL, Spitzer RL. Using the Patient Health Questionnaire-9 to measure depression among racially and ethnically diverse primary care patients. *J. Gen. Intern. Med.* 2001;16:606–13.

[40] Spitzer RL, Kroenke K, Williams JB. Validation and utility of a self-report version of PRIME-MD: the PHQ primary care study. Primary care evaluation of mental disorders. Patient Health Questionnaire. *JAMA* 1992;282:1737–44.

[41] Spitzer RL, Williams JB, Kroenke K, Hornyak R, McMurray J. Validity and utility of the PRIME-MD patient health questionnaire in assessment of 3000 obstetric-gynecologic patients: the PRIME-MD Patient Health Questionnaire Obstetrics–Gynecology Study. *Am. J. Obstet. Gynecol.* 2000;183:759–69.

[42] Martin A, Rief W, Klaiberg A, Braehler E. Validity of the brief patient health questionnaire mood scale (PHQ-9) in the general population. *Gen. Hosp. Psychiatry* 2006;28:71–7.

[43] Pinto-Meza A, Serrano-Blanco A, Penarrubia MT, Blanco E, Haro JM. Assessing depression in primary care with the PHQ-9: can it be carried out over the telephone? *J. Gen. Intern. Med.* 2005;20:738–42.

[44] Andrews G, Slade T. Interpreting scores on the Kessler psychological distress scale (K10). *Aust. NZJ Public Health* 2001;25:494–7.

[45] Aldworth J, Chromy JR, Foster M, Heller D, Novak S; RTI International. National Survey on Drug Use and Health: serious psychological distress report. Rockville, MD: Substance Abuse and Mental Health Services Administration; 2004 Available at http:// www.oas.samhsa.gov/ nsduh/2k4MRB/2k4spd.pdf. Accessed July 1, 2011.

[46] CDC. Health-related quality of life and activity limitations—eight states, 1995. *MMWR* 1998;47:134–40.

[47] Kindig DA, Asada Y, Booske B. A population health framework for setting national and state health goals. *JAMA* 2008;299:2081–3.

[48] Moriarty DG, Zack MM, Kobau R. The Centers for Disease Control and Prevention's healthy days measures—population tracking of perceived physical and mental health over time. *Health Qual Life Outcomes* 2003;2:1:37.

[49] Andresen EM, Catlin TK, Wyrwich KW, Jackson-Thompson J. Retest reliability of surveillance questions on health-related quality of life. *J. Epidemiol. Community Health* 2003;57:339–43.

[50] Kapp JM, Jackson-Thompson J, Petroski GF, Schootman M. Reliability of health-related quality-of-life indicators in cancer survivors from a population-based sample, 2005, BRFSS. *Public Health* 2009; 123:321–5.

[51] Dominick KL, Ahern FM, Gold CH, Heller DA. Relationship of health-related quality of life to health care utilization and mortality among older adults. *Aging Clin. Exp. Res.* 2002;14:499–508.

[52] Lewis G, Booth M, Regional differences in mental health in Great Britain. *J. Epidemiol. Community Health* 1992;46:608–11.

[53] Strine TW, Dhingra SS, Kroenke K, Qayad M, Ribble JL, Okoro CA. Metropolitan and micropolitan statistical area estimates of depression and anxiety using the Patient Health Questionnaire-8 in the 2006 Behavioral Risk Factor Surveillance System. *Int. J. Public Health* 2009; 54:117–24.

[54] Wardenaar KJ, Vreeburg SA, Veen TV, et al. Dimensions of depression and anxiety and the hypothalamo-pituitary-adrenal axis. *Biol. Psychiatry* 2010;15:366–73.

[55] Albert CM, Chae CU, Rexrode KM, Manson JE, Kawachi I. Phobic anxiety and risk of coronary heart disease and sudden cardiac death among women. *Circulation* 2005;111:480–7.

[56] Kawachi I, Colditz GA, Ascherio A, et al. Prospective study of phobic anxiety and risk of coronary heart disease in men. *Circulation* 1994;89: 1992–7.

[57] Kroenke K, Spitzer RL, Williams JBW, Monahan PO, Lo B. Anxiety disorders in primary care: prevalence, impairment, comorbidity, and detection. *Ann. Intern. Med.* 2007;146:317–25.

[58] Spitzer RL, Kroenke K, Williams JB, et al. A brief measure for assessing generalized anxiety disorder: the GAD-7. *Arch. Intern. Med.* 2006; 166:1092–7.

[59] Hu SS, Balluz L, Battaglia MP, Frankel MR. The impact of cell phones on public health surveillance. Bull World Health Organ 2010;77:799.

[60] Kubzansky LD, Koenen KC. A prospective study of posttraumatic stress disorder symptoms and coronary heart disease in women. *Health Psychol.* 2009;28:125–30.

[61] Aiello AE, Simanek AM, Galea S. Population levels of psychological stress, herpesvirus reactivation and HIV. *AIDS Behav.* 2010;14:308–17.

End Notes

1 Additional information available at http://www.cdc.gov/brfss/index.htm.
2 Additional information available at http://apps.nccd.cdc.gov/brfss.
3 Additional information available at http://apps.nccd.cdc.gov/brfss-smart/ index.asp.
4 Additional information available at http://apps.nccd.cdc.gov/brfss-smart/ selquickviewchart.asp.
5 Additional information available at http://apps.nccd.cdc.gov/gisbrfss/default.aspx.
6 Additional information available at http://www.cdc.gov/brfss/technical_ infodata/surveydata.htm.
7 Additional information available at http://www.cdc.gov/brfss/smart/ technical_infodata.htm.
8 Additional information available at http://www.cdc.gov/brfss/maps/gis_data.htm.
9 Additional information available at http://www.cdc.gov/nchs/nhis.htm.
10 Additional information available at http://www.cdc.gov/rdc.
11 Demographic, questionnaire, examination, and laboratory data sets are available at http://www.cdc.gov/nchs/nhanes/nhanes2007-2008/nhanes07_08.htm.
12 Additional information available at http://www.cdc.gov/prams.
13 Additional information available at http://www.cdc.gov/prams/ CPONDER.htm.
14 Additional information available at http://www.cdc.gov/nchs/ahcd.htm.
15 Additional information available at http://www.cdc.gov/nchs/nhds.htm.
16 Additional information available at http://www.cdc.gov/nchs/nnhs.htm.

INDEX

E

F

Q

R

S

T

U

V

W

Y